Low Cholesterol Desserts!

p 2 & 3, 5

Low Cholesterol Desserts!

Terri J. Siegel

The Crossing Press Specialty Cookbook Series Edited by Andrea Chesman

✳ The Crossing Press • Freedom • California 95019

They say the days go by quickly when they are filled with love, contentment, and wonderful memories . . .

This book is dedicated to those in my life who have hastened the pace: to my husband Michael, who makes my life good and gives me reason to celebrate season to season; and to my children, Jennifer and Brian, who keep my heart happy.

My heartfelt thanks to Andrea Chesman, my editor, for her knowledge, patience, and encouragement.

Library of Congress Cataloging-in-Publication Data

Siegel, Terri J.
    Low cholesterol desserts! / Terri J. Siegel.
        p. cm. — (The Crossing Press specialty cookbook series)
    Includes index.
    ISBN 0-89594-442-1 (cloth) :   ISBN 0-89594-441-3 (pbk.)
        1. Low-cholesterol diet—Recipes.   2. Desserts.   I. Title.   II. Series.
RM237.75.S47 1990
641.5'638—dc20

                                      90-40535
                                        CIP

Preface

This book grew out of my love of baking and concern for my family's health, both of which are a part of my heritage from my mother. To me, baking for family and friends is a way of both giving and receiving pleasure, so it's doubly rewarding.

Having spent the last seventeen years working in the health field as a pharmacy technician, I am fortunate to have been alerted years ago to the dangers of too much cholesterol and saturated fats in our diets. I have incorporated this valuable knowledge into planning my children's diet since the day they were born. My children, ages 16 and 6, have had the early advantages of acquiring a healthier taste for foods because of this.

A healthy approach to desserts doesn't mean you have to give up favorite recipes. Heart-healthy desserts can be just as delicious and appealing as heart-risky ones; all it takes is a little imagination and creative ingredient substitution.

This is a cookbook for everyone. We usually think of excess cholesterol as a problem that affects only adults; unfortunately, that's not the case. According to the American Academy of Pediatrics, children over the age of two should derive no more than 30 to 40 percent of their calories from fat.

Each recipe in this book has been analyzed for its nutritional content using *The Food Processor II, Nutrition of Diet Analysis System* computer software from ESHA Research. Values are given for calories, grams of saturated fats, grams of total fats, and milligrams of cholesterol that each serving contains. But what makes a recipe low cholesterol? Recent FDA guidelines for labeling commercial products establishes that a product may be labeled "cholesterol-free" if it contains less than 2 milligrams of cholesterol per serving. A product may be labeled "low-cholesterol" if it contains not more than 20 milligrams per serving. Many of the recipes contained here could be labeled "cholesterol-free"; all can be labeled low in cholesterol.

Here's another way of looking at the values given with each recipe: The American Heart Association recommends that you limit your daily cholesterol intake to 100 milligrams for each 1000 calories consumed, not to exceed 300 milligrams a day. A person on a low-cholesterol diet should limit cholesterol intake to 100 milligrams per day.

Substitution is the key to staying within the recommended limits: safflower margarine instead of butter, low-fat or skim milk instead of whole milk, lower fat cheeses, low-fat or non-fat yogurt instead of sour cream.

This cookbook is for all dessert lovers concerned about their health and eating habits. The recipes are not "diet" recipes. Instead, they introduce a way to prepare old favorites and create new favorites healthfully.

I grew up in a home with a fantastic cook—my mother. So naturally I love good food, which includes desserts. To me, a meal is really not complete until dessert has been served. Many of the recipes in this cookbook are treasures from the past, family recipes handed down from my grandmother to my mother, and then to me. I have simply updated them for today's healthy lifestyle, by cutting down or eliminating the cholesterol—but not the old-time flavor.

Contents

1
Ingredients

When adjusting your recipes to accommodate a healthier diet, it is important to remember that cholesterol keeps company with saturated fat. A diet high in saturated fat stimulates the body's production of cholesterol. Conversely, a diet that limits your cholesterol is one that is low in saturated fat.

Saturated fats are found primarily in foods of animal origin and normally are solid or firm at room temperature; for example, butter, egg yolks, whole milk or cream, lard, chocolate, and palm and coconut oils. Commercially prepared baked goods are usually loaded with saturated fat—shortening, hydrogenated oils, palm kernel oils, and coconut oil are all to be avoided.

Safflower oil is the most unsaturated of the unsaturated oils. For this reason, I use safflower oil in each recipe that calls for cooking oil. Other heart-healthy oils can be substituted, such as corn, sunflower, and soybean. Canola oil, derived from the rapeseed plant, and containing about half monounsaturates and a third polyunsaturates, is also excellent for baked goods. For several years, monounsaturates were believed to be neutral, neither raising nor lowering blood cholesterol. But recent research suggests that monounsaturates definitely assist in the lowering of cholesterol when used in place of saturated fats in the diet. Olive oil, another heart-healthy, monounsaturated oil, is too strongly flavored for use in desserts.

An easy way to distinguish between a saturated (harmful) fat and an unsaturated (safe) fat is that saturated fats (ie., butter, lard, vegetable shortening) are hard at room temperature. A good example of this can be seen in stick margarine; if it were not hydrogenated (saturated), it would not remain hard at room temperature. For this reason, I substitute tub-style safflower margarine in all recipes that call for butter or margarine. "Light" versions contain far more water than regular tub margarine and should not be used.

I use tub margarine to grease my baking pans, unless the recipe notes otherwise. Many low-cholesterol, low-fat cookbooks recommend the use of cooking spray oils for greasing pans. I have avoided them in my cooking because aerosol sprays have been implicated in the destruction of the protective ozone layer in the upper atmosphere. The manufacturers of PAM® cooking spray reported to me that PAM® does not contain any CFCs or HCFCs, the specific chemical compounds that are implicated in destroying the ozone layer. They also mentioned that they manufacture a spray oil that comes in a pump can; unfortunately, that product is not available in all areas. So use the product you feel most comfortable with—oil sprays or tub margarine—but don't forget the ozone layer!

Eggs are another ingredient that require substitution. One large egg yolk contains approximately 250 to 275 milligrams cholesterol, virtually the entire daily allowance. Therefore, whole eggs should be limited to three per week, including those found in baked goods. Luckily, exchanging whole eggs with egg substitutes—egg whites, which contain no cholesterol, commercial egg substitute, or the egg substitute recipe given in this cookbook—is easy, and the results are much the same, without the added cholesterol.

I have also replaced whole milk and cream with healthier alternatives. There is a significant difference between whole and skim milk: whole milk gets 49 percent of its calories from fat, 2 percent milk gets 35 percent of its calories from fat, whereas skim milk gets a scant 0.04 percent calories from fat.

In preparing recipes that originally used baking chocolate squares, I simply use 3 tablespoons cocoa powder plus 1 tablespoon safflower oil for each ounce of baking chocolate. Cocoa powder—the dried and pulverized liquid of the cocoa bean—has half or more of the cocoa butter removed. Unlike baking chocolate, cocoa powder contains no saturated fat.

Table of Substitutions for Healthier Cooking

The following table gives heart-healthy substitutes for fat-loaded ingredients frequently found in dessert recipes. Use the substitutes to modify your family recipes.

1 whole egg
- Egg substitute (p. 6)
- 2 egg whites plus 2 teaspoons safflower or canola oil (per whole egg)
- Commercially prepared egg substitute

1 cup whole milk
- 1 cup skim milk mixed with 1 cup instant non-fat dry milk
- Commercially prepared cholesterol-free non-dairy creamer
- 1 cup skim milk plus 2 tablespoons safflower oil

1 cup evaporated milk
- 1 cup evaporated skim milk (can be used as a whipped topping, but it should be chilled or it won't whip properly)

1 cup whole milk yogurt
- 1 cup plain non-fat yogurt

1 cup buttermilk
- Heat 1 cup skim milk to room temperature, then add 1 tablespoon lemon juice or vinegar; let stand for 5 minutes; stir

1 cup sour cream
- 1 cup plain non-fat yogurt

1 ounce baking chocolate
- 3 tablespoons cocoa powder plus 1 tablespoon safflower oil

Butter, margarine, or shortening
- Equal measure tub-style safflower margarine
- Safflower oil (proportion of butter/shortening to safflower oil):
  - 1 tablespoon to $3/4$ tablespoon oil
  - $1/3$ cup to 4 tablespoons oil
  - $1/2$ cup to 6 tablespoons oil
  - $3/4$ cup to 9 tablespoons oil
  - 1 cup to 12 tablespoons oil ($3/4$ cup)

Egg Substitute

Yield: 1 large egg equivalent or ¼ cup • Calories: 109 per recipe • Saturated Fat: 0.84 g • Total Fat: 9.11 g • Cholesterol: 0.56 mg

This will stay fresh in the refrigerator for one week, or it can be frozen for several weeks. The recipe makes the equivalent of one large egg, but it can easily be multiplied.

1 egg white
2¼ teaspoons instant non-fat dry milk
2 teaspoons safflower oil

Combine the ingredients in a blender and blend thoroughly.

Creamy Whipped Topping

Yield: 6 servings (3 cups) • Calories: 635 per recipe • Saturated Fat: 0.34 g; Total Fat: 0.58 g • Cholesterol: 12 mg

This is a light, flavorful, and heart-healthy version of whipped cream.

1 cup instant non-fat dry milk
1 cup ice water
1½ tablespoons lemon juice
1 teaspoon vanilla extract
½ cup sugar

In a small, chilled bowl, and using an electric mixer set on medium-high speed, beat the dry milk powder and ice water together until peaks form, about 5 minutes. Add the lemon juice and vanilla and continue beating until stiff. Fold in the sugar. Serve immediately.

2
Cakes

We love to celebrate with cakes. Some of our happiest memories revolve around wedding cakes, anniversary cakes, and, of course, birthday cakes.

In the following pages, you'll find recipes for chocolate cakes, layer cakes, cupcakes, and upside-down cakes, as well as a variety of toppings to complement this most traditional of desserts.

This chapter contains several variations of angel food cake, a cake that is virtually cholesterol-free. To ensure a light, cloud-like cake, you need to understand how to handle egg whites. To begin with, egg whites should increase their volume seven to eight times when beaten. This is best accomplished when using an unlined copper bowl and a wire whisk. Copper has a useful, yet harmless chemical property that binds with the albumin in the egg white, making it less likely to deflate. A stainless steel bowl is also a good choice, but don't use glass or porcelain bowls, as the egg whites will slip down the sides. The easiest way to beat the egg whites is with a heavy-duty standing mixer. If you use a hand-held mixer, you'll have to work a little harder because the egg white mixture may be deeper than the length of the beaters. In that case, use an up-and-down motion while beating (lifting the beaters from the bottom to the center of the bowl) to make sure that all of the egg whites get an equal share of the beating.

It is very important to bring the egg whites to room temperature before beating them. This usually takes about an hour, but it is well worth the time as they will beat up fuller and fluffier, producing a much higher cake. Separate the whites from the yolk when the eggs are still cold; it's much easier then.

I find that using aluminum cake pans with a dull finish work best for cake baking. One item that I found indispensable in baking both cakes and cookies is parchment paper. It can be found with paper supplies in supermarkets or in cookware stores. Parchment paper is worth its weight in gold when baking cakes: It can easily be cut into shapes for lining cake pans, therefore eliminating the step of greasing and flouring the pans, and the cakes will unmold with ease. If parchment paper is not available, waxed paper will also do the trick. Let the cakes cool for 5 to 10 minutes before removing them from the pans. Don't remove the paper until the cake is completely cooled. If you are also greasing the pan, use tub-style margarine.

Instead of using plain sugar in cakes and frostings, I cut fresh vanilla beans into 2-inch pieces and place them in my sugar canister to enhance the flavor. And always use real vanilla extract, not the imitation, when baking. The flavor is much more intense and aromatic.

The nutritional analysis of each cake recipe in this chapter includes frostings, if the frosting is listed in the ingredients list. If the frosting is merely a serving suggestion mentioned in the recipe introduction, it is not included in the analysis. Calories and other values given for cake recipes are given per serving.

Golden Layer Cake

❖❖

Yield: 12 servings, each with: Calories: 361 • Saturated Fat: 2.66 g • Total Fat: 15.4 g • Cholesterol: 0.33 mg

This light cake gets a lovely, crusty top like that of angel food cake. So I like to serve it with the top up and no frosting, beyond a garnish of fresh fruit. But it's also delicious inverted and frosted with the Fudge Frosting (page 169).

1 (8-ounce) container tub-style
   margarine
2 cups sugar
1 cup skim milk
1½ cups all-purpose flour
1 cup cornstarch
1 tablespoon baking powder
½ teaspoon salt
7 egg whites

Preheat the oven to 350° F. Line two 9-inch cake pans with parchment or waxed paper, or grease with tub-margarine and dust with cake flour.

In a large mixing bowl, beat the margarine for about 1 minute on medium speed. Add the sugar and beat thoroughly. Blend in the milk on low. Mix in the flour, cornstarch, baking powder, and salt; blend well.

In a separate mixing bowl, using clean beaters, beat the egg whites until stiff peaks form. Fold the egg whites into the batter, blending well.

Pour the batter into the cake pans, and bake for 25 to 30 minutes, or until a tester inserted near the center of the cake comes out clean. The top will become somewhat

◆◆◆

cracked. Remove the pans from the oven, and cool for 10 minutes on wire racks; then invert the cakes onto wire racks to finish cooling out of the pans. Carefully peel off the waxed paper.

To serve plain, turn the cake top side up and serve warm. Or, finish cooling the layers and frost with Fudge Frosting.

Yellow Chiffon Cake

❖❖❖

Yield: 8 servings, each with: Calories: 344 • Saturated Fat: 0.98 g • Total Fat: 10.2 g • Cholesterol: 0.55 mg

As a sheet cake, this luscious Yellow Chiffon makes a perfect base for fresh fruits. As a layer cake, try it topped with the Chocolate Meringue Frosting (page 171).

2 egg whites
1¼ cups sugar
2¼ cups all-purpose flour
1 tablespoon baking powder
½ teaspoon salt
⅓ cup safflower oil
1 cup skim milk
1 teaspoon vanilla extract
¼ teaspoon lemon extract
½ cup egg substitute (see page 6)

Preheat the oven to 350° F. Linc two 8-inch layer cake pans or one 9-inch by 13-inch baking pan with parchment or waxed paper, or grease with tub-style margarine and lightly dust with cake flour. In a small mixing bowl, beat the egg whites until frothy, gradually adding ½ cup of the sugar. Continue beating until the egg whites are stiff. Set aside.

In a large mixing bowl, sift together the remaining ¾ cup sugar, the flour, baking powder, and salt. Add the oil, ½ cup of the milk, and the vanilla and lemon extracts. Beat for 1 minute on medium speed. Add the remaining ½ cup milk and the egg substitute. Beat for 1 minute longer. Gently fold in the egg whites.

❖❖

Bake in the prepared cake pans, 30 to 35 minutes for layer cake, 40 to 45 minutes for a sheet cake, or until a tester inserted near the center of the cake comes out clean. Remove from the oven and invert onto a wire cooling rack. When completely cooled, carefully remove the parchment or waxed paper.

Fudge Cake

Yield: 8 servings, each with: Calories: 965 • Saturated Fat: 5.31 g • Total Fat: 44.5 g • Cholesterol: 1.42 mg

This moist, dark cake is low in cholesterol, but not low in calories. A good percentage of the calories comes from the frosting; so instead of using frosting to sandwich the layers, fill the layers with sliced berries. Fudge frosting can cover the top.

4 cups cake flour
2½ cups sugar
1 cup unsweetened cocoa powder
½ teaspoon cinnamon
½ teaspoon salt
2 tablespoons baking soda
1⅓ cups safflower oil
2 cups skim milk
2 cups strong, hot coffee
1 teaspoon vanilla extract
Fudge Frosting (page 169)

Preheat the oven to 350° F. Line two 8-inch cake pans with parchment or waxed paper, or grease with tub-style margarine and dust with unsweetened cocoa powder.

In a large mixing bowl, blend together the flour, sugar, cocoa, cinnamon, salt, and baking soda. Add the safflower oil and milk, and stir well. Blend in the hot coffee. Pour the batter into the cake pans and bake for 35 to 40 minutes, or until a tester inserted in the center of the cake comes out clean. Remove from the oven and invert onto a wire rack to cool. When completely cooled, carefully remove the parchment or waxed paper and top with Fudge Frosting.

Nutty Chocolate Cake

❖◆◆◆❖

Yield: 16 servings, each with: Calories: 217 • Saturated Fat: 0.92 g • Total Fat: 6.68 g • Cholesterol: 0.02 mg

1 cup all-purpose flour
½ cup whole wheat flour
1 teaspoon baking powder
½ teaspoon baking soda
¾ cup sugar
3 tablespoons unsweetened cocoa
  powder
1 teaspoon cinnamon
½ teaspoon salt
1 cup water
2 tablespoons safflower oil
2 teaspoons vanilla extract
1 teaspoon cider vinegar
¼ cup egg substitute (see page 6)
¼ cup chopped unsalted peanuts

Preheat the oven to 350° F.

In an 8-inch square ungreased baking pan, mix together the flours, baking powder, baking soda, sugar, cocoa, cinnamon, and salt. Make a well in the center of the mixture.

In a small bowl, combine the water, safflower oil, vanilla, vinegar, and egg substitute. Stir well and add to the dry ingredients. Mix until well blended. Sprinkle the chopped peanuts on top.

Bake for 30 minutes, or until a tester inserted at the center comes out clean. Cool completely in the pan on a wire rack, then frost, if desired, or serve plain.

Buttermilk-Cocoa Cake

✦✦

Yield: 8 servings, each with: Calories: 354 • Saturated Fat: 1.29 g • Total Fat: 10.1 g • Cholesterol: 1.03 mg

A rich and dense chocolate cake. A dusting of powdered sugar through a paper lace doily laid atop will transform this simple cake into a showpiece.

2 cups all-purpose flour
1½ cups sugar
2 tablespoons instant non-fat dry milk
1 teaspoon baking soda
1 teaspoon baking powder
½ teaspoon salt
½ cup water
⅓ cup safflower oil
¼ cup unsweetened cocoa powder
¾ cup low-fat buttermilk
2 egg whites
1 teaspoon vanilla extract
Powdered sugar

Preheat the oven to 350° F. Line a 9-inch square baking pan with parchment or waxed paper, or grease with tub-style margarine and lightly dust with cocoa powder.

In a large mixing bowl, sift together the flour, sugar, instant milk, baking soda, baking powder, and salt.

In a small saucepan, combine the water, oil, and cocoa. Stir and heat to boiling over a low heat. Boil for 30 seconds. Allow the mixture to cool for 10 minutes, and then add the cocoa to the flour mixture and mix until smooth. Add the buttermilk, egg whites, and vanilla, and beat for about 2 minutes at medium speed.

Pour the batter into the baking pan. Bake for 30 to 35 minutes, or until a tester inserted in the center comes out clean. The

❖❖

cake should spring back when touched in the center. Invert the cake onto a wire rack and cool completely. Carefully remove the parchment or waxed paper and top with a dusting of powdered sugar.

Marble Cake

Yield: 12 servings, each with: Calories: 314 • Saturated Fat: 1.75 g • Total Fat: 9.49 g • Cholesterol: 0.35 mg

This is one of the richest yet lightest cakes I've ever baked. The Mocha Icing is the perfect added indulgence.

3½ cups cake flour
½ teaspoon baking soda
2½ teaspoons baking powder
½ teaspoon salt
½ cup tub-style margarine, at room temperature
¾ cup sugar
¼ cup egg substitute (see page 6)
1 cup skim milk mixed with 1 teaspoon cider vinegar
1 teaspoon vanilla extract
1 tablespoon unsweetened cocoa powder

1 tablespoon sugar
1 teaspoon cinnamon
⅛ teaspoon cloves
⅛ teaspoon baking soda
1 tablespoon tub-style margarine, melted
4 egg whites
Mocha Icing (page 171)

Preheat the oven to 375° F. Grease a 10-inch tube pan with tub-style margarine.

Stir together the cake flour, baking soda, baking powder, and salt; set aside.

In a large mixing bowl, cream together the ½ cup margarine and the ¾ cup sugar; mix in the egg substitute.

Add the flour mixture, the milk and

vinegar mixture, and the vanilla. Mix thoroughly, until the batter is smooth.

In a small mixing bowl, combine the cocoa, the remaining 1 tablespoon sugar, the cinnamon, cloves, and baking soda; stir in the melted margarine. Measure out 1 cup of the cake batter and blend into the cocoa mixture; set aside.

Beat the egg whites on high speed until they are stiff, but not dry. Fold about 2/3 of the beaten egg whites into the plain cake batter and the remaining third into the cocoa batter.

Pour the plain batter into the tube pan. Drop generous spoonfuls of the cocoa batter onto the plain batter, swirling the cocoa batter through the plain. Bake for 30 minutes, or until a tester inserted in the center comes out clean. Invert the cake onto a wire rack and cool completely. Frost with Mocha Icing when it has cooled.

Angel Food Cake

❖❖❖

Yield: 12 servings, each with: Calories: 157 • Saturated Fat: 0.01 g • Total Fat: 0.07 g • Cholesterol: 0 mg

Because it contains no fat or cholesterol, angel food cake always makes a light, refreshing dessert. Try serving it doused with Strawberry Sauce (page 168) and garnished with mint, or frost it lightly with Buttercream Icing (page 170).

1½ cups sifted powdered sugar
1 cup sifted cake flour
1½ cups egg whites (10 to 12 large eggs), at room temperature
1½ teaspoons cream of tartar
1 teaspoon vanilla extract
1 cup sugar

Preheat the oven to 350° F.

Sift the powdered sugar and cake flour together 3 times; set aside.

Beat together the egg whites, cream of tartar, and vanilla on medium speed until soft peaks form (the tips will curl). Gradually add the sugar, about 2 tablespoons at a time, now beating on high speed until stiff peaks form (the tips will stand straight).

Sift about ¼ of the flour mixture over the beaten egg whites and very gently fold it in. Repeat this step of sifting over and folding in the remaining flour mixture 3 more times.

Pour the batter into an ungreased 10-inch tube pan. Using a metal spatula or butter knife, cut through the batter to release any large air pockets. Place the cake in the

❖❖

center of the lowest rack of the oven to give it room to rise. Baking in the center of the oven will insure even browning.

Bake for 40 to 45 minutes, or until the top of the cake springs back when lightly touched. The crust of the cake should be a golden brown and slightly cracked.

Remove the cake from the oven and immediately invert the tube pan. Cool the cake completely before turning upright. Loosen the sides of the cake and carefully remove from the pan. To serve, use a serrated knife to slice the cake into wedges.

Chocolate Angel Food Cake

❖❖❖

Yield: 12 servings, each with: Calories: 124 • Saturated Fat: 0.21 g • Total Fat: 0.4 g • Cholesterol: 0 mg

Try the Sweet Cherry Sauce (page 168) with this version. The combination of chocolate and cherry is truly fit for angels.

¾ cup sifted cake flour
¼ cup unsweetened cocoa powder
¼ teaspoon cinnamon
1¼ cups sugar
12 egg whites, at room temperature
1 teaspoon cream of tartar
¾ teaspoon vanilla extract
¾ teaspoon almond extract
Powdered sugar

Preheat the oven to 350° F.

Sift together the cake flour, cocoa, cinnamon, and ¼ cup of the sugar; set aside.

In a large mixing bowl, beat the egg whites until they are foamy; add the cream of tartar, and continue to beat at high speed until the whites are stiff. Gradually fold in the remaining cup of sugar with a rubber spatula; do the same with the extracts. When blended, fold in the flour mixture gently.

Spread the batter into an ungreased 10-inch tube pan. Place the cake in the center of the lowest rack of the oven, and bake for 45 minutes, or until the top of the cake springs back when lightly touched. The crust of the cake should be a golden brown and slightly cracked.

❖❖

After removing from the oven, immediately invert the cake pan. Cool thoroughly before carefully loosening the cake from the sides of the pan and then removing the pan. To serve, dust the top with sifted powdered sugar, and slice the cake into wedges with a serrated knife.

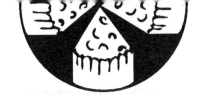

Fruited Cocoa Angel Cake

❖❖❖

Yield: 12 servings, each with: Calories: 207 • Saturated Fat: 0.3 g • Total Fat: 0.7 g; • Cholesterol: 0 mg

This is an elegant variation that combines the taste of chocolate and fresh fruit. Peaches make a delicious substitute for the nectarines.

Cake

1½ cups sifted powdered sugar
1 cup sifted cake flour
⅓ cup unsweetened cocoa powder
½ teaspoon ground ginger
1½ cups egg whites (10 to 12 large
   eggs), at room temperature
1½ teaspoons cream of tartar
1 teaspoon vanilla extract
1 cup sugar

Nectarine Sauce

3 (5½-ounce) cans peach nectar
3 tablespoons cornstarch
2 tablespoons water
1 tablespoon minced crystallized ginger
   root
1 teaspoon grated lemon rind
¾ teaspoon lemon juice
¼ teaspoon vanilla extract
3 nectarines, sliced (do not peel)

Preheat the oven to 350° F.

Sift the powdered sugar, cake flour, cocoa, and ginger together 3 times; set aside.

Beat together the egg whites, cream of tartar, and vanilla on medium speed until soft peaks form (the tips will curl). Gradually add the sugar, about 2 tablespoons at a time, beating on high speed until stiff peaks form (the tips will stand straight).

Sift about ¼ of the flour mixture over the beaten egg whites and fold in very gently. Repeat this step of sifting over and folding in the remaining flour mixture 3 more times.

Pour the batter into an ungreased 10-inch tube pan. Using a metal spatula or butter knife, cut through the batter to release any large air pockets. Place the cake in the center of the lowest rack of the oven, and bake for 40 to 45 minutes, or until the top springs back when lightly touched. The crust should be slightly cracked and golden brown.

Remove the cake from the oven and immediately invert the pan. Cool the cake completely before turning upright. Loosen the cake from the sides of the pan and carefully remove the pan.

In a medium-size saucepan, heat the peach nectar until hot. In a small cup, blend the cornstarch with the water until smooth; add to the peach nectar, stirring constantly. Simmer until thickened. Remove from the heat and stir in the crystallized ginger root, lemon rind, lemon juice, and vanilla. Cool the mixture for 5 minutes. Stir in the nectarine slices.

To serve, slice the cooled cake with a serrated knife and top each slice with a generous helping of the warm nectarine sauce.

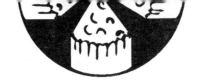

Coffee-Marble Angel Food Loaf

❖❖

Yield: 8 servings, each with: Calories: 186 • Saturated Fat: 0.23 g • Total Fat: 0.45 g • Cholesterol: 0 mg

You can skip the Mocha Icing and top it with a scoop of ice milk and fresh berries if you prefer.

½ cup cake flour
Dash salt
¾ cup sugar
5 egg whites, at room temperature
½ teaspoon cream of tartar
½ teaspoon vanilla extract
2 teaspoons instant coffee powder
Mocha Icing (page 171)

Preheat the oven to 375° F.

Sift together the cake flour, salt, and ¼ cup of the sugar. Set aside.

Beat the egg whites, cream of tartar, and vanilla until peaks form. Gradually fold in the flour. Pour ⅔ cup of the batter into an ungreased 10-inch loaf pan. Gently stir the instant coffee into the remaining batter and spread this mixture over the plain batter. With a sweeping, folding motion, combine the batters just enough to give a marbled effect.

Bake for 25 minutes, or until the top springs back when lightly touched. Invert the cake onto a wire rack and cool completely in the pan. Loosen the sides of the cake from the pan and carefully remove the pan. Frost with Mocha Icing.

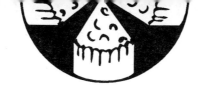

Blueberry Cake

Yield: 9 servings, each with: Calories: 247 • Saturated Fat: 1.82 g • Total Fat: 10.8 g • Cholesterol: 0.13 mg

This flavorful cake is perfect for a mid-morning coffee break. Serve warm, dusted with white sugar.

½ **cup tub-style margarine, at room temperature**
½ **cup sugar**
¼ **cup egg substitute (see page 6)**
¼ **cup skim milk**
2 **cups all-purpose flour**
2½ **teaspoons baking powder**
¼ **teaspoon salt**
1 **teaspoon cinnamon**
½ **teaspoon vanilla extract**
1 **cup blueberries, fresh or frozen and drained after rinsing**
2 **teaspoons sugar**

Preheat the oven to 350° F.

Grease an 8-inch square baking pan with tub-style margarine.

In a medium-size mixing bowl, mix together the margarine, ½ cup sugar, and egg substitute until well blended. Add the milk. Stir in the flour, baking powder, salt, cinnamon, and vanilla, and mix thoroughly. Fold in the blueberries until they are just coated.

Spread the batter evenly into the pan and bake for 35 to 40 minutes, or until a tester inserted in the center comes out clean. Dust with the remaining 2 teaspoons sugar while still warm.

Peach Cake

❖❖

Yield: 9 servings, each with: Calories: 201 • Saturated Fat: 1.3 g • Total Fat: 7.73 g • Cholesterol: 0.26 mg

Crunchy streusel topping baked on top of a rich peach-filled shortcake.

Cake

1½ cups all-purpose flour
2½ teaspoons baking powder
½ teaspoon salt
¼ teaspoon nutmeg
⅓ cup tub-style margarine, at room temperature
½ cup sugar
½ cup egg substitute (see page 6)
½ teaspoon vanilla extract
½ teaspoon almond extract
1 teaspoon lemon zest
½ cup skim milk
2 medium-ripe peaches, peeled, sliced

Topping

1 tablespoon sugar
⅛ teaspoon cloves
⅛ teaspoon cinnamon
⅛ teaspoon nutmeg

Preheat the oven to 375° F. Grease an 8-inch square baking pan with tub-style margarine.

Mix together the flour, baking powder, salt, and nutmeg; set aside.

In a large mixing bowl, beat the margarine, sugar, and egg substitute on medium speed until light. Add the vanilla and almond extracts and the lemon zest. Add the flour mixture along with the milk, and beat until thoroughly blended.

Spread the batter evenly into the baking

pan. Arrange the peach slices on top of the batter. Mix together the ingredients for the topping, and sprinkle over the peach slices.

Bake for 35 to 40 minutes, or until a tester inserted in the center comes out clean. The flavor is best when the cake is served warm.

Caramel-Apple Cake

Yield: 9 servings, each with: Calories: 414 • Saturated Fat: 2.08 g • Total Fat: 17.9 g • Cholesterol: 0.3 mg

A very moist cake, dense with apples, deliciously topped with a rich caramel sauce.

Cake

1 cup packed dark brown sugar
½ cup safflower oil
2 teaspoons cinnamon
1 tablespoon vanilla extract
¼ cup egg substitute (see page 6)
1 egg white
2 cups all-purpose flour
½ teaspoon salt
1 tablespoon baking powder
2 medium-size cooking apples, coarsely
    chopped (do not peel)

Caramel Topping

½ cup packed light brown sugar
¼ cup tub-style safflower margarine
¼ cup skim milk
2 tablespoons non-fat dry milk
1 teaspoon vanilla extract

Preheat the oven to 350° F. Grease a 9-inch square baking pan with tub-style margarine.

In a large mixing bowl, beat together the brown sugar, safflower oil, cinnamon, and vanilla. Add the egg substitute and the egg white; beat well. Mix in the flour, salt, and baking powder, just until blended. Stir in the apples.

Pour the batter into the baking pan and bake for 30 to 40 minutes, or until the cake

◆◆◆

springs back when touched in the center.

To make the topping, stir together the brown sugar, margarine, skim milk, and powdered milk in a small saucepan; bring to a boil. Lower the heat and simmer, stirring for about 5 minutes, or until thickened. Remove from heat and stir in the vanilla. Pierce the entire surface of the hot cake with a fork and pour the caramel topping over the cake. Serve the cake warm.

Pineapple Upside-Down Cake

❖❖

Yield: 8 servings, each with: Calories: 473 • Saturated Fat: 2.77 g • Total Fat: 16.4 g • Cholesterol: 0.18 mg

A traditional American favorite. I add a hint of rum flavoring to the tender cake.

Topping

3 tablespoons tub-style margarine, melted
1 cup packed light brown sugar
1 (20-ounce) can crushed pineapple, packed in juice

Cake

½ cup tub-style margarine, at room temperature
1 cup sugar
2 egg whites
¼ cup egg substitute (see page 6)

1½ cups all-purpose flour
2 teaspoons baking powder
¼ teaspoon salt
½ teaspoon vanilla extract
½ teaspoon rum extract
Enough evaporated skim milk mixed with the reserved pineapple juice to make ¾ cup liquid

Preheat the oven to 350° F.

To prepare the topping, pour the melted margarine into a 9-inch deep-dish pie plate. Spread the brown sugar evenly over the butter. Drain the pineapple; save the liquid (you will need this for the cake batter). Arrange the pineapple on the brown sugar. Set aside.

In a large mixing bowl, combine the margarine, sugar, egg whites, and egg substitute; cream until light and fluffy. Add the remaining ingredients, and beat for 2 minutes until the batter is smooth. Spoon the batter evenly over the pineapple-brown sugar mixture. Bake for 50 to 55 minutes, or until the edges of the cake begin to brown and a tester inserted in the center of the cake comes out clean. Remove from the oven and cool the cake in the pan on a wire rack for 5 minutes. Carefully invert the cake onto a cake plate. Serve warm or cold.

Blueberry Upside-Down Cake

Yield: 9 servings, each with: Calories: 397 • Saturated Fat: 2.23 g • Total Fat: 14.9 g • Cholesterol: 0.35 mg

This upside-down cake contains oat flour, which has a nut-like flavor. Oat flour can be found in health food stores or in the health food aisle of your supermarket. If the flour is unavailable, simply grind a couple of tablespoonfuls of rolled oats in the blender to a fine powder.

Topping

2 cups blueberries, fresh or frozen and
    drained after rinsing
½ cup sugar
2 tablespoons oat flour
2 tablespoons lemon juice

Cake

½ cup tub-style margarine, at room
    temperature
1 cup sugar
2 egg whites
¼ cup egg substitute (see page 6)
¾ cup skim milk
2 cups all-purpose flour
4 teaspoons baking powder
½ teaspoon salt
1 teaspoon almond extract
1 tablespoon grated lemon zest
½ cup toasted slivered almonds

Preheat the oven to 350° F. Grease a 9-inch springform pan.

To prepare the topping, gently toss all the ingredients together in a medium-size mixing bowl and mix well; spread the mixture evenly in the pan. Set aside.

In a large mixing bowl, beat the margarine, sugar, and egg whites on medium speed for about 2 minutes. Add the egg substitute, milk, flour, baking powder, salt, and almond extract. Beat for 1 minute, until thoroughly smooth. Stir in the lemon zest. Pour the batter over the berry mixture in the prepared pan.

Bake for 70 minutes, or until a tester inserted in the center of the cake comes out clean. Remove the sides of the pan and invert the cake onto a cake platter. Carefully remove the bottom of the pan, and arrange the almonds decoratively over the berries.

Note: To toast the almonds, heat a dry 8-inch skillet over medium heat. Add the almonds and cook for 5 to 6 minutes, stirring frequently until they are golden brown. Remove from the heat and cool.

Carrot-Pineapple Cake

◆◆

Yield: 10 servings, each with: Calories: 650 • Saturated Fat: 3.25 g • Total Fat: 30.2 g • Cholesterol: 0.29 mg

This hearty old-fashioned cake is moist and full of fruit.

2 cups all-purpose flour
1 cup packed light brown sugar
2 teaspoons baking powder
1 teaspoon cinnamon
½ teaspoon baking soda
¼ teaspoon salt
3 cups grated carrots
⅔ cup safflower oil
⅔ cup skim milk
¼ cup egg substitute (see page 6)
1 cup crushed pineapple, well drained
½ cup raisins
1 cup chopped pecans
Creamy Pineapple Frosting (page 172)

Preheat the oven to 350° F. Line two 8-inch layer cake pans with parchment or waxed paper, or grease with tub-style margarine and lightly dust with flour.

In a medium-size mixing bowl, combine the flour, brown sugar, baking powder, cinnamon, baking soda, and salt. Add the carrots, oil, milk, egg substitute, pineapple, raisins, and pecans; blend very well.

Pour into the prepared pans and bake for 30 to 35 minutes, or until a tester inserted in the center comes out clean. Cool the layers in the pans on wire racks for 5 minutes. Invert onto the wire racks and cool completely before removing the paper linings.

Frost the cooled layers with Creamy Pineapple Frosting.

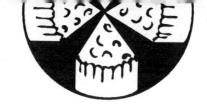

Pumpkin Cake

Yield: 12 servings, each with: Calories: 533 • Saturated Fat: 3.2 g • Total Fat: 34.6 g • Cholesterol: 0.05 mg

Dense and moist, this cake is spicy and not too sweet. Try a slice with fresh fruit for breakfast.

2 cups all-purpose flour
2 cups sugar
2 cups canned or cooked and pureed
   pumpkin
1⅓ cups safflower oil
1½ cups chopped walnuts
2 teaspoons baking powder
1 teaspoon baking soda
½ teaspoon salt
½ cup egg substitute (see page 6)
2 teaspoons pumpkin pie spice
2 tablespoons powdered sugar

Preheat the oven to 350° F. Grease a 10-inch tube or bundt pan with tub-style margarine and dust with flour.

Combine all of the ingredients, except the powdered sugar, in a large mixing bowl. Blend well on medium speed for 2 minutes.

Pour the batter into the pan and bake for 1 hour, or until a tester inserted in the center of the cake comes out clean. Cool the cake completely on a wire rack before removing from the pan. To serve, invert the cooled cake onto a cake plate and lightly sift powdered sugar over the top.

Rum-Topped Applesauce Cake

Yield: 12 servings, each with: Calories: 739 • Saturated Fat: 4.28 g • Total Fat: 33.8 g • Cholesterol: 0.83 mg

This makes a delicious, fruity, firm-texture cake. The flavors are heartily complemented by the rum topping.

Cake
¾ cup safflower oil
1¾ cups sugar
2 cups unsweetened applesauce
1 tablespoon baking soda
¾ cup raisins
¾ cup chopped walnuts
3½ cups sifted all-purpose flour
1 tablespoon unsweetened cocoa
   powder
¼ teaspoon salt
¾ teaspoon cinnamon
¾ teaspoon allspice

Rum Topping
1 cup tub-style margarine
1 cup evaporated skim milk
2 cups sugar
2 teaspoons vanilla extract
2 tablespoons dark rum

Preheat the oven to 350° F. Generously grease a 10-inch tube pan with tub-style margarine and dust with cocoa.

In a large mixing bowl, combine the safflower oil and sugar. Stir in the applesauce and baking soda. Add the raisins and chopped walnuts.

Stir together the flour, cocoa, salt, cinnamon, and allspice. Blend into the applesauce mixture, and beat for 1 to 2 minutes, or until the batter is well blended.

Pour the batter into the tube pan and bake for 1 hour, or until a tester inserted in the center comes out clean. Remove the cake from the oven, place on a wire rack, and let cool completely in the pan before inverting it onto a cake plate.

To prepare the Rum Topping, melt the margarine with the milk in a medium-size saucepan. Add the sugar and cook over medium heat until the sugar dissolves and the sauce begins to thicken (about 3 minutes). Remove from the heat and stir in the vanilla and the rum. To serve, place the cake slices on dessert plates and top with the warm rum topping.

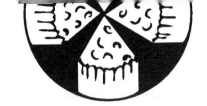

Banana-Nut Cake

❖❖❖

Yield: 12 servings, each with: Calories: 433 • Saturated Fat: 2.45 g • Total Fat: 18.1 g • Cholesterol: 0.12 mg

¾ cup tub-style margarine, at room
   temperature
1½ cups sugar
½ cup egg substitute (see page 6)
1 cup mashed bananas (2 to 3 medium-
   size bananas)
1 teaspoon vanilla extract
¼ cup non-fat plain or vanilla yogurt
2¼ cups cake flour
½ teaspoon baking powder
¾ teaspoon baking soda
¼ teaspoon salt
1 cup chopped walnuts
Brown Sugar Frosting (page 169)

Preheat the oven to 350° F. Line a 9-inch by 13-inch cake pan or two 8-inch layer cake pans with parchment or waxed paper.

Beat the margarine, sugar, and egg substitute until creamy, about 2 minutes. Add the bananas, vanilla, and yogurt; beat for 1 minute on medium speed.

Blend together the flour, baking powder, baking soda, and salt. Add bananas and beat well for 2 minutes. Stir in the chopped nuts.

Spread the batter into the cake pan(s) and bake for about 30 minutes, or until the center of the cake springs back when touched. Cool for 5 minutes in the pan(s) on a wire rack. Invert the cake onto a wire rack and cool completely before removing the paper and frosting.

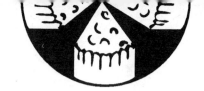

Light Lemon Cake

Yield: 9 servings, each with: Calories: 173 • Saturated Fat: 0.97 g • Total Fat: 5.91 g • Cholesterol: 0.26 mg

As the name implies, this is very light in texture. A cinnamon-sugar topping is a sweet complement to the cake's tangy flavor. I serve it warm, topped with sliced fresh strawberries.

1 cup all-purpose flour
2 teaspoons finely grated lemon rind
½ teaspoon salt
½ teaspoon baking powder
¼ cup tub-style margarine, at room
    temperature
¾ cup sugar
½ cup egg substitute (see page 6)
1 tablespoon lemon juice
½ cup skim milk
2 egg whites
Cinnamon sugar

Preheat the oven to 350° F. Grease an 8-inch square baking pan with tub-style margarine and dust with flour.

Stir together the flour, lemon rind, salt, and baking powder.

In a small mixing bowl, beat the margarine and sugar at medium speed for 2 minutes. Add the egg substitute and the lemon juice, mixing until well blended. Add the flour mixture and milk alternately to the beaten mixture, beating on low speed until just combined.

Beat the egg whites on high speed until stiff peaks form. Fold into the batter.

Pour the batter into the pan and bake for 30 to 35 minutes, or until the center of the cake springs back when touched.

Sprinkle the warm cake lightly with cinnamon sugar and serve.

Old-Fashioned Pound Cake

❖❖

Yield: 10 servings, each with: Calories: 246 • Saturated Fat: 1.84 g • Total Fat: 10.3 g • Cholesterol: 1.18 mg

This cake is not only delicious, it is versatile as well. Serve it plain or top with Blueberry Sauce (page 169). Yogurt in the batter gives the cake a rich taste. You can experiment with flavored yogurts to give it a slightly different flavor.

⅔ cup sugar

½ cup tub-style margarine, at room temperature

½ cup egg substitute (see page 6)

1 tablespoon vanilla extract

1 teaspoon almond extract

2½ cups sifted cake flour

¾ teaspoon baking soda

¼ teaspoon salt

1 (8-ounce) carton low-fat vanilla yogurt

Preheat the oven to 350° F. Using tub-style margarine, grease a 9-inch x 5-inch loaf pan, then lightly dust with cake flour.

Cream the sugar and tub margarine at medium speed until light and fluffy. Add the egg substitute and beat for 4 minutes. Add the vanilla and almond extracts; beat at low speed until well blended. With the mixer running at low speed, add the flour, baking soda, and salt to the creamed mixture. Add the yogurt, and blend well.

Pour the batter into the prepared loaf pan and bake for 65 minutes, or until a tester inserted in the center of the cake comes out clean. Cool in the pan on a wire rack for 10 minutes; remove from the pan and finish cooling the cake on a wire rack. Serve plain or topped with fruit.

Nectarine Pound Cake

❖❖❖

Yield: 10 slices, each with: Calories: 359 • Saturated Fat: 2.6 g • Total Fat: 14.7 g • Cholesterol: 1.02 mg

2 tablespoons all-purpose flour
2 tablespoons packed light brown sugar
2 nectarines, peeled and sliced
¾ cup tub-style margarine, at room temperature
1 cup white sugar
2½ cups all-purpose flour
½ teaspoon baking soda
1 teaspoon baking powder
½ teaspoon salt
1 teaspoon vanilla extract
1 (8-ounce) carton non-fat lemon yogurt
¼ cup egg substitute (see page 6)
1 egg white

Preheat the oven to 325° F. Grease a 10-inch bundt pan with margarine, dust with flour.

Blend the 2 tablespoons flour and brown sugar together; add the nectarines and toss until well coated. Place this mixture in the bottom of the prepared bundt pan.

In a large bowl, beat the margarine and white sugar. Blend in 2½ cups flour, baking soda, baking powder and salt. Add the vanilla, yogurt, egg substitute, and egg white; beat for 3 minutes at medium speed.

Pour the batter over the nectarine mixture and bake for 1 hour, or until a tester inserted in the center of the cake comes out clean.

Remove the cake and cool in the pan for 10 minutes. Invert onto a wire rack and cool completely before serving.

43

Lemon-Blueberry Pound Cake

◆◆

Yield: 8 serving, each with: Calories: 307 • Saturated Fat: 2.04 g • Total Fat: 11.9 g • Cholesterol: 0.5 mg

When blueberries are in season, this lemon-spiced pound cake is irresistible topped with Blueberry Sauce (page 169).

⅔ cup sugar
½ cup tub-style margarine, at room
    temperature
3 egg whites
2 teaspoons vanilla extract
1 teaspoon lemon extract
2½ cups sifted cake flour
¾ teaspoon baking soda
½ teaspoon salt
1 (8-ounce) carton non-fat plain yogurt
1½ teaspoons grated lemon zest
1 cup fresh blueberries

Preheat the oven to 350° F. Grease an 8-inch loaf pan with tub-style margarine and lightly dust with cake flour.

In a large mixing bowl, cream the sugar, margarine, and egg whites; beat for 4 minutes at medium speed, or until well blended. Add the vanilla and lemon extracts; beat at low speed until blended.

Combine the flour, baking soda, and salt; gradually add to the creamed mixture alternately with the yogurt. Stir in the lemon zest. Gently fold in the blueberries.

Pour the batter into the prepared loaf pan and bake for 65 minutes, or until a tester inserted in the center comes out clean. Cool for 10 minutes. Remove the cake from the pan and finish cooling on a wire rack.

Cocoa-Walnut Pound Cake

◆◆

Yield: 8 servings, each with: Calories: 365 • Saturated Fat: 2.98 g • Total Fat: 17.9 g • Cholesterol: 1.47 mg

This extra-rich version of the classic pound cake is a chocolate lover's dream. Add a few slices of fresh strawberries on top, and you're set for anything.

2½ cups sifted cake flour
⅔ cup sugar
⅓ cup unsweetened cocoa powder
½ cup tub-style margarine, at room temperature
½ cup egg substitute (see page 6)
1 tablespoon vanilla extract
1 teaspoon almond extract
¾ teaspoon baking soda
¼ teaspoon salt
1 (8-ounce) carton non-fat vanilla yogurt
½ cup chopped walnuts

Preheat the oven to 350° F. Grease an 8-inch loaf pan with tub-style margarine and lightly dust with cocoa powder.

Sift together the cake flour, sugar, and cocoa; set aside.

In a large mixing bowl, combine the margarine, egg substitute, and vanilla and almond extracts; beat for 4 minutes on medium speed.

Add the flour mixture; blend well. Mix in the baking soda and salt. Add the yogurt and blend thoroughly. Stir in the chopped walnuts.

Pour into the loaf pan and bake for 60 to 65 minutes. Cool the pound cake in the pan for 10 minutes; remove from the pan and cool on a wire rack. Top with fresh fruit if desired.

Gingerbread with Lemon Sauce

✦✦

Yield: 12 servings, each with: Calories: 262 • Saturated Fat: 1.37 g • Total Fat: 8.15 g • Cholesterol: 0.02 mg

Add warmth to a crisp fall afternoon with the luscious aroma and taste of gingerbread. Made with molasses, this gingerbread is wonderfully spicy.

Gingerbread

1 cup boiling water
½ cup tub-style margarine
1 cup light molasses
2½ cups all-purpose flour
⅓ cup sugar
1 teaspoon baking soda
½ teaspoon salt
1 teaspoon ground ginger
½ teaspoon cinnamon
½ teaspoon ground cloves
¼ cup egg substitute (see page 6)

Lemon Sauce

⅓ cup sugar
4 teaspoons cornstarch
1 cup cold water
½ teaspoon lemon zest
2 tablespoons lemon juice

Preheat the oven to 350° F. Lightly grease a fluted 10-inch tube pan with tub-style margarine and dust with flour.

In a large mixing bowl, pour the boiling water over the margarine, stirring to melt the margarine. Stir in the molasses.

Stir together the flour, sugar, baking soda, salt, ginger, cinnamon, and cloves. Gradually add to the molasses mixture; beat lightly only until blended. Add the egg

❖❖

Variation: Yield: 9 servings, each with: Calories: 526 • Saturated Fat: 2.71 g • Total Fat: 16 g • Cholesterol: 0.24 mg.

substitute, and beat until smooth.

Pour the batter into the greased tube pan and bake for 45 to 50 minutes, or until the center of the cake springs back when lightly touched. Remove from the oven and cool in the pan on a wire rack for 10 minutes. Invert the cake onto a wire rack and cool.

To make the sauce, combine the sugar, cornstarch, and cold water in a small saucepan. Cook and stir over medium heat until thickened and bubbly; cook 2 minutes longer. Remove from the heat and stir in the lemon zest and the lemon juice. Cover with waxed paper and cool.

To serve, place a slice of cake on each dessert plate, top with Creamy Whipped Topping (page 6), if desired, and the lemon sauce over the cream.

Gingerbread with Butterscotch Pear Sauce

Prepare the gingerbread as in previous recipe, but bake the cake in a greased and floured 9-inch square baking pan. Instead of the lemon sauce, prepare the Butterscotch Pear Sauce by mixing together 1 cup packed light brown sugar, ½ cup light corn syrup, ¼ cup tub-style margarine, and ½ cup skim milk in a medium-size saucepan. Cook over low heat for 5 minutes, stirring occasionally. Stir in 2 teaspoons lemon zest and 1 (16-ounce) can sliced pears, drained. Heat through. Spoon the sauce over the gingerbread squares.

Chocolate Zucchini Snack Cake

Yield: 16 servings, each with: Calories: 139 • Saturated Fat: 0.86 g • Total Fat: 7.68 g • Cholesterol: 0.16 mg

This is a great dessert that packs well: perfect for lunch boxes.

2½ cups all-purpose flour
2 teaspoons baking powder
½ teaspoon baking soda
¼ teaspoon salt
2 cups, grated, unpeeled zucchini
¼ cup unsweetened cocoa powder
1 teaspoon cinnamon
½ cup safflower oil
¼ cup non-fat buttermilk
2 teaspoons vanilla extract
½ cup egg substitute (see page 6)
Powdered sugar

Preheat the oven to 350° F. Grease a 9-inch by 13-inch baking dish with tub-style margarine.

In a large mixing bowl, combine all the ingredients except the powdered sugar. Stir until thoroughly blended.

Pour the batter into the baking dish and bake for 45 minutes, or until a tester inserted in the center of the cake comes out clean. Cool completely in the pan on a wire rack. Dust with powdered sugar before cutting into bars.

Cocoa Orange Cupcakes

◆◆

Yield: 12 cupcakes, each with: Calories: 144 • Saturated Fat: 0.76 g • Total Fat: 6.53 g • Cholesterol: 0.17 mg

These are absolutely the best chocolate cupcakes I've ever tasted—bursting with the wonderful flavor combination of chocolate and orange. They are also easily made in one bowl, with no mixer required.

1 cup all-purpose flour
⅔ cup sugar
¼ cup unsweetened cocoa powder
¾ teaspoon baking soda
½ teaspoon grated orange zest
¼ teaspoon salt
½ cup skim milk
½ cup orange juice
⅓ cup safflower oil
Sifted powdered sugar

Preheat the oven to 350° F. Line 12 muffin cups with paper liners.

In a large mixing bowl, stir together the flour, sugar, unsweetened cocoa powder, baking soda, orange zest, and salt. Combine the milk, orange juice, and oil; stir into the dry ingredients. Beat by hand until well blended. The batter will be fairly thin.

Pour the batter into the muffin cups, filling the cups ⅔ full. Bake for 30 to 35 minutes. When done, the cupcakes should spring back when lightly touched in the center. Remove the cupcakes from the tin and cool on a wire rack. Top with sifted powdered sugar.

Spice Cupcakes

❖❖

Yield: 10 cupcakes, each with: Calories: 205 • Saturated Fat: 0.85 g • Total Fat: 4.76 g • Cholesterol: 0.2 mg

These aromatic cupcakes will make your kitchen smell heavenly as they bake.

1 cup all-purpose flour
1¼ teaspoons baking powder
¼ teaspoon salt
¼ teaspoon ginger
½ teaspoon nutmeg
½ teaspoon cinnamon
¼ cup tub-style margarine, at room temperature
⅔ cup sugar
1¼ teaspoons vanilla extract
½ cup skim milk
2 egg whites
Vanilla Glaze (page 171)

Preheat the oven to 375° F. Line 10 muffin cups with paper liners.

In a medium-size mixing bowl, stir together the flour, baking powder, salt, ginger, nutmeg, and cinnamon; set aside.

Beat together the margarine, sugar, and vanilla; continue beating for 2 minutes. Add the dry ingredients alternately with the milk; mix thoroughly on medium speed.

Beat the egg whites on medium speed until stiff peaks form. Fold the beaten egg whites into the flour mixture.

Fill the muffin cups ⅔ full. Bake for 15 to 20 minutes, or until the top bounces back when lightly touched. Remove the cupcakes from the tin and cool on a wire rack. Frost lightly with Vanilla Glaze.

50

3
Pies and Tarts

Pies and tarts are at their best when they are simple and homey. I've had a long-standing love affair with flaky pastries filled with fruits or fillings and, fortunately, a lighter version of pastry is just as flaky as a fat-ladened pastry and quite simple to make.

The trick to making successful pastry is to not overmix, or the finished product will become tough. The less you handle the dough the better. It is always a good idea to refrigerate the pastry dough for at least half an hour before rolling it out. When you're ready to roll out the dough, use a floured rolling pin on a lightly floured surface. Move the dough around to make a circle, always working from the center out to the edges. Fold the dough in half and carefully ease it into the pie pan. Unfold the dough and crimp the edges (for a single-crust pie). For a double-crust pie, fill the bottom crust, place the second crust over the filling, fold over the two edges, and then crimp. Sprinkle 1 to 2 teaspoons of sugar over the top crust before baking.

Tart shells differ from pie crusts in that they must be able to stand on their own when removed from the pan. The shells can be made with a flaky pastry dough or a meringue. The free-standing Meringue Nut Crust filled with seasonal fresh fruit produces an impressive looking (and tasting) dessert, but be sure not to grind the nuts. Oil is released from nuts when they're ground, and the presence of oil breaks down the meringue.

I have included several pie shell pastries so that you can choose the best one to enhance the filling you've selected.

The nutritional analysis of each pie and tart recipe includes the pastry crust, but does not include whipped or ice milk toppings; these are extras, added at your own discretion. The nutritional analysis for the pastry crust recipes are figured per serving.

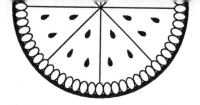

Cherry Pie

◆◆

Yield: 8 servings, each with: Calories: 357 • Saturated Fat: 2.02 g • Total Fat: 11.8 g • Cholesterol: 0 mg

This treasured recipe was handed down from my great-grandmother to my mother, and then to my sister and me. Use a deep-dish pie pan if you have one available, and top with a lattice crust if you have the time.

1 recipe Flaky Pastry (page 72)
1¼ cups sugar
3 tablespoons cornstarch
2 (16-ounce) cans tart, pitted cherries (in juice)
½ teaspoon almond extract
¼ teaspoon cinnamon

Prepare the pastry according to the recipe directions. Line a 9-inch pie pan with the bottom crust. Keep the top crust refrigerated.

Preheat the oven to 400° F.

In a saucepan, combine the sugar and cornstarch. Add the cherries and juice. Cook over medium heat, stirring constantly until thickened; boil for 1 minute. Remove from the heat; stir in the almond extract and cinnamon. Pour into the pastry-lined pie pan.

Roll out the top crust and cover the pie. Flute the edges together and cut several slashes in the top crust for steam. Or cut the top crust into strips and weave a lattice top.

Bake for 10 minutes, reduce the heat to 350° F., and continue baking for 30 minutes longer. Cool before slicing—the filling will firm up as it cools.

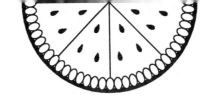

Fresh Berry Pie

Yield: 8 servings, each with: Calories: 357 • Saturated Fat: 2.02 g • Total Fat: 11.8 g • Cholesterol: 0 mg

Any berry will do for this pie. Top it with a generous scoop of ice milk for a delicious summer treat.

1 recipe Flaky Pastry (page 72)
2 tablespoons all-purpose flour
½ cup sugar
¼ teaspoon salt
4 cups fresh berries (strawberries, blueberries, or blackberries)
1 teaspoon lemon juice
¼ teaspoon almond extract
1 teaspoon sugar

Prepare the pastry according to the recipe directions. Line a 9-inch pie pan with the bottom crust.

Preheat the oven to 450° F.

In a large bowl, mix together the flour, ½ cup sugar, and salt; sprinkle ¼ of the mixture on the bottom crust. Coat the berries with the lemon juice and almond extract, then toss them with the remaining sugar mixture.

Pour the berries into the pie plate. Roll out the top crust and fit over the berries; crimp the edges. Prick the top crust to allow steam to escape and sprinkle with the remaining 1 teaspoon sugar.

Bake for 15 minutes; reduce the heat to 350° F., and continue baking for another 25 to 30 minutes. Cool the pie before serving.

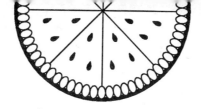

Apple Pie

Yield: 8 servings, each with: Calories: 413 • Saturated Fat: 2.56 g • Total Fat: 15.0 g • Cholesterol: 0 mg

When my mother used to make this pie, I had the job of tasting the cinnamon-apple slices to approve the spicing. My 6-year-old was fortunate to inherit this position.

1 recipe Flaky Pastry (page 72)
1 cup sugar
2 teaspoons cinnamon
8 to 9 tart apples (Pippins are
   recommended), peeled and thinly sliced
2 tablespoons all-purpose flour
2 tablespoons tub-style margarine
1 teaspoon sugar

Prepare the pastry according to the recipe directions. Line a 9-inch pie pan with the bottom crust. Preheat the oven to 425° F.

Mix together the sugar and cinnamon; toss with the apples until the slices are well coated. Arrange in the pastry-lined pie plate. Sprinkle the flour and dot with the margarine.

Roll out the top crust and fit over the apples; crimp the edges. Make a few decorative air vents and sprinkle the top of the crust with the remaining 1 teaspoon sugar.

Bake for 15 minutes; reduce the oven temperature to 350° F., and continue baking the pie for another 50 to 55 minutes. If the crust starts to brown too quickly, cover the crust edges with foil. Cool the pie for 20 minutes before serving.

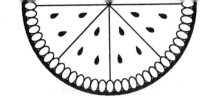

Apple Cranberry Pie

❖❖

Yield: 8 servings, each with: Calories: 415 • Saturated Fat: 2.58 g • Total Fat: 15.0 g • Cholesterol: 0 mg

Apple and cranberries make a particularly pleasing contribution—both to the eye and to the palate. I keep plenty of frozen cranberries on hand so I can serve this pie year-round.

1 recipe Flaky Pastry (page 72)
¾ cup packed light brown sugar
¼ cup white sugar
⅓ cup all-purpose flour
¾ teaspoon cinnamon
⅛ teaspoon nutmeg
4 to 5 baking apples, pared and sliced
2 cups fresh or frozen cranberries
2 tablespoons tub-style margarine
1 teaspoon sugar

Prepare the pastry according to the recipe directions. Line a 9-inch pie pan with the bottom crust.

Preheat the oven to 425° F.

In a large bowl, stir together the brown sugar, ¼ cup white sugar, the flour, cinnamon, and nutmeg. Add the apple slices and the cranberries; toss to coat the fruit well. Pour the fruit mixture into a pastry-lined pie plate; dot with the margarine.

Roll out the top crust and fit over the pie; flute the edges. Cut decorative slits in the top crust to release steam and sprinkle with the remaining 1 teaspoon of sugar. Bake for 40 minutes. Cool before serving. Top with ice milk, if desired.

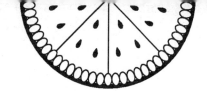

Apple Rhubarb Pie

Yield: 8 servings, each with: Calories: 378 • Saturated Fat: 2.52 g • Total Fat: 14.8 g • Cholesterol: 0 mg

The pungent rhubarb complements the smooth apples in this pie.

1 recipe Flaky Pastry (page 72)
1 cup sugar
⅓ cup all-purpose flour
¼ teaspoon salt
½ teaspoon cinnamon
2 cups rhubarb, cut into 1-inch pieces
3 cups sliced baking apples
2 tablespoons tub-style margarine
1 tablespoon lemon juice
½ teaspoon sugar

Prepare the pastry according to the recipe directions. Line a 9-inch pie pan with the bottom crust.

Preheat the oven to 400° F.

In a large mixing bowl, combine the sugar, flour, salt, and cinnamon. Toss with the rhubarb and apples. Spoon the mixture into a pastry-lined pie plate. Dot with margarine and sprinkle with lemon juice.

Roll out the top crust and fit on the pie; seal and flute the edges. Cut decorative slits in the top for steam. Sprinkle the crust with the remaining ½ teaspoon sugar. Bake for 55 minutes. Cool before slicing.

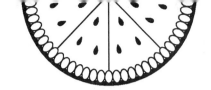

French Apple Pie

Yield: 8 servings, each with: Calories: 458 • Saturated Fat: 3.08 g • Total Fat: 17.9 g • Cholesterol: 0 mg

Pie

½ recipe Flaky Pastry (page 72)
¾ cup sugar
¼ cup all-purpose flour
½ teaspoon nutmeg
¼ teaspoon cinnamon
6 to 7 baking apples, peeled and thinly
  sliced (about 6 cups)

French Crumb Topping

1 cup all-purpose flour
½ cup tub-style margarine
½ cup packed light brown sugar

Prepare the pastry according to the recipe directions. Line a 9-inch pie pan with the pastry. Trim and flute the edges.

Preheat the oven to 375° F.

In a large mixing bowl, mix the sugar, flour, nutmeg, and cinnamon. Toss the apples with the flour mixture until the apples are well coated. Pour the apples into the pastry-lined pie plate.

In a small mixing bowl, combine all the topping ingredients with a pastry blender or 2 knives until the mixture is crumbly. Sprinkle the topping evenly over the apples.

Bake for 40 minutes, cover the topping with foil, and continue baking for 10 more minutes. Remove the pie from the oven and let set for 5 minutes before serving.

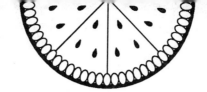

Pumpkin Pie

Yield: 8 servings, each with: Calories: 273 • Saturated Fat: 1.21 g • Total Fat: 6.97 g • Cholesterol: 1.71 mg

½ recipe Flaky Pastry (page 72)
2 cups canned or cooked and pureed pumpkin
½ cup white sugar
½ cup packed light brown sugar
½ cup egg substitute (see page 6)
2 egg whites
¼ teaspoon salt
1 tablespoon pumpkin pie spice
1 (12-ounce) can evaporated skim milk

Prepare the pastry according to the recipe directions. Line a 9-inch pie pan with the pastry. Trim and flute the edges.

Preheat the oven to 400° F.

In a large mixing bowl, combine all the remaining ingredients. Beat at medium speed until smooth, about 3 minutes. Pour into the unbaked pie shell. Bake for 10 minutes, then reduce the oven temperature to 325° F., and bake for 50 minutes more, or until a knife inserted at the center comes out clean. Serve either warm or chilled, with a generous helping of Creamy Whipped Topping (page 6). Refrigerate any leftover pie.

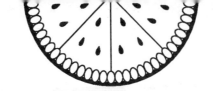

Fresh Peach Pie

◆◆◆

Yield: 8 servings, each with: Calories: 292 • Saturated Fat: 0.87 g • Total Fat: 13.4 g • Cholesterol: 0 mg

Full of fresh peaches and flavored with orange rind on top, this no-bake pie served in a Meringue Nut Crust makes a delightful summertime dessert.

Meringue Nut Crust (page 71)
7 medium-size ripe peaches
¾ cup orange juice
¾ cup sugar
3 tablespoons cornstarch
2 tablespoons lemon juice
2 teaspoons finely grated orange zest

Prepare the pie shell according to the recipe directions. Bake and set aside to cool.

Peel and slice enough peaches to make 1 cup. Puree the peaches in a blender, adding the orange juice as it is being pureed.

In a medium-size saucepan, blend the sugar with the cornstarch. Add the peach puree and mix well. Bring the mixture to a boil over medium high heat, stirring constantly. Cool the puree quickly by setting the pan in cold water; stir frequently until only slightly warm.

Peel and slice the remaining peaches; toss with the lemon juice. Gently stir the peach slices into the puree, then pour the mixture into the cooled pie shell. Chill until cool, about 45 minutes. Before serving, garnish the pie with the grated orange zest.

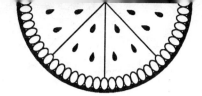

Fresh Strawberry Pie

Yield: 8 servings, each with: Calories: 265 • Saturated Fat: 1.32 g • Total Fat: 9.67 g • Cholesterol: 0 mg

Fresh whole strawberries are folded into an almond-flavored puree and baked in an oatmeal crust. Top it with a generous helping of the Creamy Whipped Topping (page 6), if you like.

Prebaked Oatmeal Pie Crust (page 74)
¾ cup sugar
3½ tablespoons cornstarch
5 cups strawberries, washed and hulled
½ cup water
¼ teaspoon almond extract

Prepare the pie shell according to the recipe directions. Bake and set aside to cool.

In a 3-quart saucepan, mix together the sugar and cornstarch. Mash 2 cups of the strawberries. Add the mashed strawberries and the water to the sugar mixture. Cook over medium heat, stirring constantly, until the mixture comes to a boil; reduce the heat and boil gently for 2 minutes. Remove from the heat and stir in the almond extract. Let cool. Fold the remaining strawberries into the cooled mixture. Pour into the prepared pastry shell and chill for at least 1 hour before slicing.

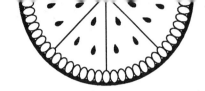

Banana Cream Pie

❖❖

Yield: 8 servings, each with: Calories: 404 • Saturated Fat: 2.58 g • Total Fat: 14.8 g • Cholesterol: 1.5 mg

This creamy pie tastes so rich, it's hard to believe you're eating a low-fat, low-cholesterol version.

1 prebaked 9-inch pie shell (pages 71–74)
2¼ cups water
1 cup instant non-fat dry milk
¾ cup sugar
2 egg whites, beaten
¼ cup cornstarch
¼ teaspoon salt
2 tablespoons tub-style margarine
2 teaspoons vanilla extract
2 large bananas (not overly ripe), sliced
2 egg whites
¼ teaspoon cream of tartar
¼ cup sugar

Prepare the pie shell according to the recipe directions. Bake and set aside to cool.

Preheat the oven to 425° F.

In a medium-size saucepan, combine the water, instant non-fat milk, ¾ cup sugar, beaten egg whites, cornstarch, and salt. Simmer over a low heat, stirring constantly until thickened. Continue cooking and stirring for 2 minutes longer. Remove from the heat and add the margarine and vanilla. Stir lightly until the margarine has melted; cool. Add the banana slices, and pour the filling into the pie shell.

In a small mixing bowl, combine the remaining 2 egg whites and cream of tartar and beat until frothy. Gradually add the remaining ¼ cup sugar, beating at high speed to form a meringue. Spread on the pie, making sure to seal the edges of the crust with meringue so that it will not shrink while baking.

Bake for 8 to 10 minutes, or until lightly browned. Let the pie cool completely on a wire rack, and then refrigerate.

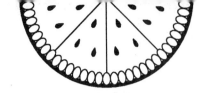

Lemon Chiffon Pie

❖❖

Yield: 8 servings, each with: Calories: 230 • Saturated Fat: 0.86 g • Total Fat: 13.3 g • Cholesterol: 0 mg

Be sure to chill the filling before spooning it into the Meringue Nut Crust—it will mound higher and produce a fluffier pie. For a special touch, sprinkle the top with grated crystallized ginger.

Meringue Nut Crust (page 71)
1 tablespoon gelatin
¼ cup cold water
½ cup sugar
¼ cup boiling water
½ cup lemon juice
1 teaspoon grated lemon zest
¼ teaspoon salt
3 egg whites
½ cup corn syrup

Prepare the pie shell according to the recipe directions. Bake and set aside to cool.

In a small bowl, stir together the gelatin and cold water; let the gelatin soften for about 5 minutes. Mix in the sugar and boiling water until the sugar and gelatin are dissolved. Stir in the lemon juice and zest. Chill the mixture just until it is syrupy. Do not let it set or the finished product will not be smooth.

In a medium-size mixing bowl, beat the salt and the egg whites until stiff. Beating continually, gradually add the corn syrup. Fold in the lemon mixture, then chill for 20 minutes. Spoon the mixture into the meringue shell and chill until set.

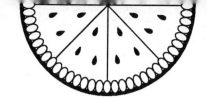

French Apple Tart

Yield: 8 servings, each with: Calories: 147 • Saturated Fat: 1.05 g • Total Fat: 6.1 g • Cholesterol: 0 mg

Easily prepared and full of fruit, this spectacular dessert should be served right from the oven.

½ **recipe Flaky Pastry (page 72)**
½ **cup unsweetened applesauce**
4 baking apples, peeled and thinly sliced
2 teaspoons orange juice
¼ **teaspoon nutmeg**
Powdered sugar

Prepare the dough according to the recipe directions. On a floured surface, roll out the dough to a 12-inch circle. Fit the pastry into a 9-inch tart pan with a removable bottom. Trim and flute the edges.

Preheat the oven to 350° F.

Spread half the applesauce in the pastry shell. Begin to overlap the apple slices in a circular design, starting from the outer edge. Continue arranging the apples in a pinwheel design until the whole tart pan is covered. Sprinkle the orange juice and grated nutmeg evenly over the apples. Brush the remaining applesauce on top of the apples.

Bake for 20 to 25 minutes. When done, the apples should be golden. Sprinkle the tart with the powdered sugar and serve at once.

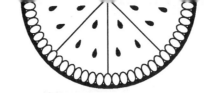

Fresh Pear Tart

❖◆❖

Yield: 8 servings, each with: Calories: 523 • Saturated Fat: 3.46 g • Total Fat: 22.4 g • Cholesterol: 1.57 mg

Here's an elegant dessert. Ground ginger spices up the filling, and crystallized ginger accents the Creamy Whipped Topping. Using red Bosc pears makes a delicious variation.

Pastry
1⅓ cups all-purpose flour
½ teaspoon sugar
6 tablespoons tub-style margarine
2 tablespoons safflower oil
2 tablespoons ice water

Filling
5 ripe Bartlett pears
2 tablespoons lemon juice
1 cup sugar
⅓ cup all-purpose flour
½ teaspoon ground ginger
¾ cup egg substitute (see page 6)
6 tablespoons tub-style margarine

Topping
Creamy Whipped Topping (page 6)
2 tablespoons minced crystallized ginger

Preheat the oven to 350° F.

In a medium-size mixing bowl, combine the flour and sugar. Add the margarine and safflower oil. With a fork, blend the mixture until it is very crumbly. Gradually add the water, stirring with the fork just until the dough leaves the sides of the bowl and can be gathered into a ball. Chill for 15 minutes for easier handling.

On a floured surface, roll out the dough to a 12-inch circle. Fit the pastry into a 9-inch tart pan with a removable bottom. Trim and flute the edges. Refrigerate.

To prepare the filling, cut the pears in half lengthwise. Peel and core the pears and place them in a bowl of water with the lemon juice. (This will help to keep the pears from turning brown while baking.)

In a small bowl, mix together the sugar, flour, ginger, and egg substitute. Melt the margarine in a small skillet over low heat until it is foamy and lightly golden. Stirring quickly, gradually beat the melted margarine into the sugar mixture.

Drain the pears and set them on a paper towel to dry. Place the pears, cut side down, on a cutting board and cut them crosswise in $\frac{1}{8}$-inch-thick slices. Carefully transfer the pear slices to the tart shell, slightly overlapping each pear with the next. Repeat this until all the pears have been sliced and fitted into the shell. Pour the sugar mixture evenly over the pears.

Place the tart pan on a baking sheet. Bake for 50 to 55 minutes, or until the tart is puffed and golden. Cool the tart completely on a wire rack. To serve, remove the tart from the pan and place it on a dessert serving tray. Prepare the Creamy Whipped Topping according to the recipe directions, folding in the crystallized ginger. Slice the tart into serving pieces and top with the whipped topping.

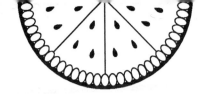

Plum Tart

Yield: 10 servings, each with: Calories: 180 • Saturated Fat: 0.85 g • Total Fat: 5.31 g • Cholesterol: 0 mg

Pastry

1 cup all-purpose flour
⅛ teaspoon salt
⅛ teaspoon sugar
⅛ teaspoon cinnamon
¼ cup tub-style margarine
4 to 6 tablespoons ice water

Filling

14 to 16 ripe red plums, cut into quarters
½ teaspoon grated lemon zest
3 tablespoons sugar
⅓ cup apricot jam
¼ teaspoon almond extract

To make the pastry, combine the flour, salt, sugar, and cinnamon. Cut the margarine into the flour until the mixture resembles coarse meal. Add the ice water a few tablespoons at a time. Mix lightly until the pastry forms into a ball. Cover and refrigerate for 30 minutes.

On a floured surface, roll out the dough to form a 10-inch by 28-inch rectangle, about ¼-inch thick. Place the dough on a baking sheet.

Preheat the oven to 400° F.

Toss the plums with the lemon zest. Arrange on the pastry, overlapping the pieces. Stop within 1 inch of the sides. Roll in the edges of the dough to meet the plums, crimping to form a ridge. Sprinkle with the sugar. Bake for 30 to 40 minutes, until the crust is crisp. Heat the jam through, stir in the almond extract, and spread it over the top of the tart. Serve warm.

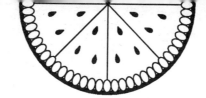

Red Grape and Almond Tart

Yield: 8 servings, each with: Calories: 305 • Saturated Fat: 1.51 g • Total Fat: 10.7 g • Cholesterol: 0.02 mg

The ground almonds in the pastry shell lend a rich, nutty flavor to the tart.

Pastry

¼ **cup egg substitute (see page 6)**
¾ **cup all-purpose flour**
½ **cup ground almonds (2 ounces)**
¼ **cup tub-style margarine, softened**
4 **teaspoons sugar**
¼ **teaspoon almond extract**

Filling

2 **cups seedless red grapes, cut in half**
1 **tablespoon unflavored gelatin**
1 **tablespoon water**
2 **tablespoons rum**
1 **(12-ounce) jar red currant jelly**

Preheat the oven to 350° F.

In a small mixing bowl, blend together all the pastry ingredients. Beat on medium speed until the pastry is crumbly and well mixed. Press onto the bottom and up the sides of a lightly oiled 9-inch tart pan. Bake the pastry for 12 to 15 minutes, or until a golden brown. Cool.

Arrange the grape halves, cut side down, on the crust. In a small saucepan, blend together the gelatin, water, and rum; let it stand for 5 minutes to allow the gelatin to soften. Stir in the jelly. Cook over medium heat, continuing to stir, until the jelly is melted and the gelatin is dissolved. Spoon the mixture over the grapes. Chill the tart for 30 minutes, or until set.

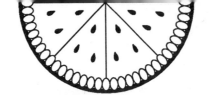

Streusel Blueberry Tarts

Yield: 8 servings, each with: Calories: 258 • Saturated Fat: 1.6 g • Total Fat: 17.4 g • Cholesterol: 0.06 mg •

Rich tasting and satisfying, these individual tarts are very easy to make, but be sure not to overfill the tarts with too many berries.

½ cups all-purpose flour
¼ teaspoon salt
⅛ teaspoon nutmeg
1 teaspoon sugar
½ cup safflower oil
2 tablespoons skim milk
1 pint fresh blueberries, washed and
    drained
¾ cup all-purpose flour
3 tablespoons sugar
2 tablespoons safflower oil
⅛ teaspoon cinnamon

Preheat the oven to 425° F.

Sift together the flour, salt, nutmeg, and sugar. Add the safflower oil and milk; beat with a fork until well blended. Divide among eight 3-inch tart pans or muffin tins. Pat the pastry onto the bottom and up the sides of the pans and fill each about ⅔ full with berries.

Toss all the remaining ingredients together until crumbly, and sprinkle the topping over the berries. Bake for 45 minutes. Cool the tarts in the pans on a wire rack for at least 15 minutes before removing from the pans. These are delicious served warm or chilled.

Page 70

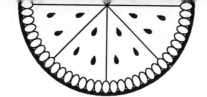

Meringue Nut Crust

❖❖

Yield: 9-inch crust • Calories: 168 • Saturated Fat: 0.85 g • Total Fat: 13.3 g • Cholesterol: 0 mg

This is a perfect prebaked pie shell for a fresh fruit or cream filling.

1 egg white
¼ cup sugar
1½ cups finely chopped nuts (not ground)

Preheat the oven to 350° F. Line a 9-inch pie plate with parchment or waxed paper.

In a small mixing bowl, beat the egg white at high speed until stiff. Gradually add the sugar while continuing to beat on high speed to form a meringue. Fold in the nuts and spread evenly in the pie plate. Be sure to smooth the meringue up around the sides of the pan.

Bake for 10 minutes. Remove from the oven and cool for a few minutes. Gently remove the crust from the pan and cool on a wire rack before filling.

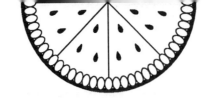

Flaky Pastry

Yield: 1 to 2 pie shells • Calories: 207 • Saturated Fat: 2.0 g • Total Fat: 11.7 g • Cholesterol: 0 mg

The nutritional analysis is based on a serving of double-crusted pie (not including any filling). Simply cut the values in half to figure out the values for a serving of single-crust pie shell.

2 cups all-purpose flour
½ teaspoon salt
¼ teaspoon sugar
½ cup tub-style margarine
7 to 9 tablespoons ice water

In a medium-size bowl, combine the flour, salt, and sugar. Using a fork, cut the margarine into the flour mixture, pressing the back of the fork against the inside of the mixing bowl. Continue doing this until the mixture resembles coarse meal. Add the ice water, a few tablespoons at a time. Mix lightly and quickly (or the dough will become tough) until the pastry forms into a ball. Divide the ball in two, and flatten each piece into a disk. Cover and refrigerate for 1 hour.

To make a double crust pie, roll out 1 disk on a lightly floured surface into a 12-inch circle. Fit into a 9-inch or 10-inch pie pan. Trim the dough to be 1 inch larger than the pan. Fill the pie as desired. Roll out the top crust and fit over the pie. Trim the dough to be slightly larger than the bottom crust. Fold the top crust over the bottom crust. Seal and crimp the edges.

To make a single crust pie or tart shell, roll out the dough on a floured surface into a 12-inch circle. Place the pastry in the pie (or tart) pan. Flute the edges.

For a prebaked pie or tart shell, prick the pie shell at $\frac{1}{4}$-inch intervals with the tines of a fork. To prevent the bottom from buckling up in the oven, line the shell with foil and fill with dried beans or pie weights. Bake in a pre-heated 400° F. oven for 10 to 15 minutes.

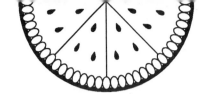

Oatmeal Pie Crust

❖❖❖

Yield: 9-inch pie shell • Calories: 156 • Saturated Fat: 1.3 g • Total Fat: 9.3 g • Cholesterol: 0 mg

1 cup rolled oats
⅓ cup packed light brown sugar
⅓ cup finely chopped walnuts
4 tablespoons tub-style margarine, melted
¼ teaspoon cinnamon
¼ teaspoon nutmeg

Preheat the oven to 375° F. Grease a 9-inch pie pan.

In a small mixing bowl, stir together the oats, brown sugar, and walnuts. Add the melted margarine, cinnamon, and nutmeg; mix well. Press the dough onto the bottom and up the sides of the pie pan. Bake for 8 to 10 minutes. Cool before filling with meringue, fresh fruit, or cream filling.

4
Fruit Desserts

Fruit desserts can range from something as simple as poached fresh fruit to impressive displays, such as Fruit-Filled Meringues or Maple-Glazed Pear Crêpes.

Fruits are naturally sweet and usually require little additional sugar. Whenever possible, use fresh fruit and be sure to freeze some fresh fruits and berries for out-of-season enjoyment. If you need to use canned fruit, make certain it is packed in juice, not syrup, and doesn't contain added sugar.

Not only are fruits nutritious, they may also help in lowering cholesterol. Research has shown that pectin, a form of soluble fiber in fruits, helps to lower high cholesterol levels. The most concentrated sources of pectin are to be found in tart apples, citrus fruits, plums, and cranberries.

For those recipes calling for fresh pineapple, look for fruit that is plump, slightly soft to the touch, devoid of bruises or mold, heavy for its size, and with deep, green leaves at the crown. An uncut pineapple can be stored in the refrigerator for up to 2 days. It's best not to leave a pineapple out at room temperature, as this will cause it to soften and lose acid. Once you have removed the rind, you can store the flesh, covered, in the refrigerator for another 1 to 2 days.

In choosing apples for making applesauce, the best ones are tart and slightly acid, such as Granny Smith, Pippin, McIntosh, and Jonathan.

Remember, the best possible natural dessert is fresh fruit, served alone or as a topping for a delicious healthful dessert you've prepared yourself.

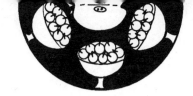

Amaretto Apples with Meringue

◆◆◆

Yield: 6 servings, each with: Calories: 110 • Saturated Fat: 0.05 g • Total Fat: 0.28 g • Cholesterol: 0 mg

⅓ cup Amaretto
½ cup water
1 tablespoon lemon juice
1 cinnamon stick
4 medium-size cooking apples, peeled
  and thinly sliced
3 egg whites
½ teaspoon grated lemon zest
3 tablespoons sugar

Preheat the oven to 325° F.

In a medium-size saucepan, combine the Amaretto, water, lemon juice, and cinnamon stick; bring to a boil. Add the apple slices and return to boiling. Reduce the heat and simmer, stirring occasionally, for 8 to 10 minutes, or until the apples are barely tender. Remove from the heat and let the apples stand in the cooking liquid for 15 minutes. Remove the cinnamon stick.

While the apples are setting, beat the egg whites in a small mixing bowl on medium speed until soft peaks form. Gradually add 1 tablespoon only of the apple cooking liquid, the lemon zest, and the sugar. Beat on the highest speed until stiff peaks form.

Divide the apple slices and the cooking liquid evenly among 6 (6-ounce) ovenproof dessert or custard cups. Top each with the egg white mixture.

Bake for about 10 minutes, or until the meringue is a light, golden brown. This is best when served warm.

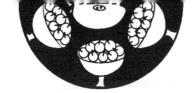

Strawberries with Meringue

❖❖

Yield: 6 servings, each with: Calories: 138 • Saturated Fat: 0.13 g • Total Fat: 1.59 g • Cholesterol: 0 mg

A cloud of soft meringue floats on warm, orange-flavored berries in this simple dessert.

2 tablespoons slivered almonds
6 cups strawberries, rinsed, hulled, and sliced
8 tablespoons sugar
¼ cup orange juice
3 egg whites
¼ teaspoon cream of tartar
1 tablespoon powdered sugar

Bake the almonds in a single layer in a pan at 350° F. for about 10 minutes, or until they are golden. Remove from the oven and increase the oven temperature to 500° F.

Mix the strawberries with 2 tablespoons of the sugar and the orange juice. Pour into a shallow 2-quart baking dish.

In a large bowl, combine the egg whites and cream of tartar; beat on high speed until foamy. Gradually add the remaining 6 tablespoons of sugar, beating just until the egg whites hold stiff, moist peaks. Mound this mixture over the center of the strawberries. Sprinkle the almonds evenly over the meringue. Sift the powdered sugar on top.

Bake just until golden, about 4 minutes. Place on dessert plates. Serve at once.

78

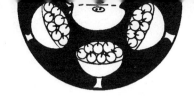

Fruit-Filled Meringues

❖❖❖

Yield: 6 servings, each with: Calories: 126 • Saturated Fat: 0.02 g • Total Fat: 0.45 g • Cholesterol: 0 mg

2 egg whites
½ teaspoon vanilla extract
⅛ teaspoon cream of tartar
½ cup sugar
3 cups strawberries, hulled and sliced
3 kiwi fruit, peeled and thinly sliced
2 tablespoons Grand Marnier

Preheat the oven to 250° F. Line a baking sheet with either parchment paper or waxed paper.

In a large mixing bowl, beat the egg whites at medium speed with the vanilla and cream of tartar until frothy. At high speed, beat in the sugar, 2 tablespoons at a time, until stiff peaks form. Spoon 6 mounds of the meringue mixture onto the baking sheet.

With a metal spatula, spread each mixture into a small rectangle shape. Place the remaining meringue in a pastry bag fitted with a star tip, and then pipe the meringue around the edge of each rectangle, making a big, decorative border.

Bake for 1 hour. Turn off the heat; let stand in the oven for 1 hour, or until dry. Set aside.

In a medium-size bowl, combine 1 cup of the strawberries with the kiwi fruit. Place the remaining strawberries and Grand Marnier in a blender. Just before serving, spoon some sauce into each meringue shell and fill each with the fruit mixture.

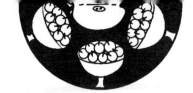

Peach Meringue Delight

❖❖

Yield: 6 servings, each with: Calories: 91 • Saturated Fat: 0.15 g • Total Fat: 1.46 g • Cholesterol: 0 mg

The taste of summer can be enjoyed any time of the year with the use of canned peaches, as in this dessert.

3 egg whites
¼ teaspoon cream of tartar
⅛ teaspoon nutmeg
¼ cup sugar
1 teaspoon almond extract
2 tablespoons ground almonds
6 canned peach halves, packed in juice and drained

Preheat the oven to 325° F. Line a cookie sheet with parchment or waxed paper.

In a small mixing bowl, beat the egg whites, cream of tartar, and nutmeg until peaks begin to form. Slowly beat in the sugar until the peaks are stiff but not dry. Fold in the almond extract and ground almonds. Using half the meringue, form 6 mounds, leaving 2 inches between each. Place a peach half on each mound, cut side up, and cover with the remaining meringue.

Bake for 30 minutes. Remove with a spatula to a wire rack and cool before serving.

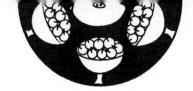

Nectarine and Plum Crisp

❖❖

Yield: 6 servings, each with: Calories: 292 • Saturated Fat: 1.82 g • Total Fat: 10.9 g • Cholesterol: 0 mg

My choice of plums for this crisp is the Santa Rosa, which has a rich, tart flavor. This is delicious served warm or cold with vanilla ice milk.

Fruit

1 pound nectarines, sliced
1 pound plums, sliced
¼ cup packed light brown sugar
¼ teaspoon cinnamon

Crisp Topping

½ cup rolled oats
⅓ cup packed light brown sugar
⅓ cup whole wheat flour
¼ teaspoon cinnamon
5 tablespoons tub-style margarine

Preheat the oven to 375° F.

In a medium-size bowl, toss the nectarines and plums with the brown sugar and cinnamon. Pour the fruit into a 9-inch pie plate.

For the topping, combine the oats, brown sugar, wheat flour, and cinnamon. Cut in the margarine with a fork until the mixture is crumbly. Sprinkle the topping evenly over the fruit.

Bake for 45 minutes. Serve warm or cold.

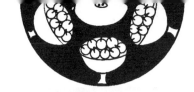

Apple Crisp

❖❖

Yield: 8 servings, each with: Calories: 256 • Saturated Fat: 0.63 g • Total Fat: 6.0 g • Cholesterol: 0 mg

I love to serve this warm with a hot cup of spicy tea. It's just as good for breakfast the next day.

6 to 7 tart cooking apples, peeled and
 sliced
1 tablespoon lemon juice
½ cup white sugar
1¼ teaspoons cinnamon
¼ teaspoon nutmeg
¾ cup rolled oats
½ cup all-purpose flour
1 cup packed light brown sugar
3 tablespoons safflower oil

Preheat the oven to 350° F.

Place the apples in a 9-inch deep-dish pie plate. Sprinkle the apples with the lemon juice, white sugar, cinnamon, and nutmeg.

In a small mixing bowl, stir together the oats, flour, brown sugar, and safflower oil; sprinkle over the apples. Bake uncovered for 40 minutes. Serve warm or cold.

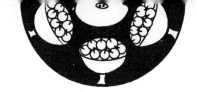

Apple Kuchen

Yield: 8 servings, each with: Calories: 301 • Saturated Fat: 2.10 g • Total Fat: 12.6 g • Cholesterol: 0.17 mg

This recipe highlights the main ingredient—apples—with the accent of peach preserves.

1¼ cups all-purpose flour
½ cup sugar
1½ teaspoons baking powder
½ cup tub-style margarine
½ cup egg substitute (see page 6)
¼ cup skim milk
1 teaspoon vanilla extract
4 to 5 cooking apples, peeled and thinly sliced
1 teaspoon cinnamon
⅓ cup low-sugar peach preserves

Preheat the oven to 400° F.

In a medium-size bowl, combine the flour, ¼ cup of the sugar, and the baking powder; mix well. Blend in ¼ cup of the margarine, the egg substitute, milk, and vanilla. Stir just until the dough sticks together. Spread the dough evenly in a 9-inch by 13-inch baking dish.

Arrange the apple slices in concentric circles on top of the dough. Melt the remaining ¼ cup margarine, and stir in the cinnamon and remaining ¼ cup of sugar. Brush this mixture over the apples.

Bake for 35 to 40 minutes. In the last 5 minutes of cooking, brush the peach preserves over the kuchen. Serve warm or cold.

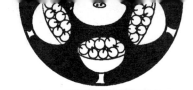

Cranapple Crunch

◆◆◆

Yield: 8 servings, each with: Calories: 261 • Saturated Fat: 1.05 g • Total Fat: 8.35 g • Cholesterol: 0 mg

A very colorful dessert. The tartness of the apples blends beautifully with the sweet, pungent cranberry sauce.

2 cups chopped unpeeled tart apples
1 (16-ounce) can whole-berry cranberry sauce
2 tablespoons tub-style margarine, melted
1 cup rolled oats
⅓ cup packed light brown sugar
¼ cup all-purpose flour
½ cup chopped walnuts

Preheat the oven to 350° F.

Combine the apples and the cranberry sauce and spread the mixture in an 8-inch square baking pan. Combine all the other ingredients and spread this over the apple-cranberry mixture.

Bake for 35 to 40 minutes. Serve warm, topped with your favorite ice milk or Creamy Whipped Topping (page 6).

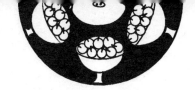

Peach Crisp

❖❖

Yield: 8 servings, each with: Calories: 239 • Saturated Fat: 1.86 g • Total Fat: 13.0 g • Cholesterol: 0 mg

I use Elberta peaches for this crisp. Select peaches that are somewhat firm. The easiest way to peel peaches is to blanch them in boiling water for almost 20 seconds, then dip them in ice water. The peel slips right off.

6 large, ripe peaches, peeled and sliced
1½ tablespoons white sugar
1 tablespoon instant tapioca
1 cup rolled oats
⅓ cup all-purpose flour
⅛ teaspoon nutmeg
¼ cup packed light brown sugar
⅓ cup tub-style margarine
½ cup chopped walnuts

Preheat the oven to 375° F.

Place the peaches in a 7-inch by 11-inch baking dish. Combine the sugar and tapioca; sprinkle over the fruit and toss well to coat.

In a small mixing bowl, combine the oats, flour, nutmeg, and brown sugar. Add the margarine and blend with a fork until the mixture is crumbly. Stir in the chopped walnuts, then sprinkle the mixture evenly over the fruit.

Bake for 35 to 40 minutes. Serve the crisp warm.

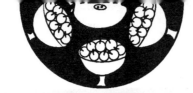

Rhubarb Cobbler

Yield: 8 servings, each with: Calories: 188 • Saturated Fat: 0.39 g • Total Fat: 3.89 g • Cholesterol: 0.25 mg

Fruit

¾ cup sugar
2 tablespoons cornstarch
1 cup water
½ cup orange juice
4 cups rhubarb, sliced into 1-inch
  pieces

Dumplings

½ cup all-purpose flour
¼ cup whole wheat flour
¼ cup rolled oats
1½ teaspoons baking powder
½ cup skim milk
2 tablespoons safflower oil
1 tablespoon sugar
¼ teaspoon cinnamon

Preheat the oven to 425° F.

In a small saucepan, stir together the ¾ cup sugar and the cornstarch. Blend in the water and orange juice. Cook and stir over medium heat until the mixture is thickened and bubbly. Add the rhubarb pieces and bring the mixture back to boiling. Remove from the heat; cover the mixture to keep it warm.

For the dumplings, stir together the flours, oats, and baking powder in a medium-size mixing bowl. Mix the milk and safflower oil together and add to the flour mixture; stir only until the flour mixture is moistened. Don't overmix.

Pour the warm rhubarb mixture into a 2-quart casserole. Quickly spoon the dump-

86

ling batter into 8 mounds on top of the warm rhubarb mixture.

In a small dish, stir together the remaining 1 tablespoon sugar and the cinnamon. Sprinkle it over the top of the dumplings.

Bake, uncovered, for about 20 minutes, or until a toothpick inserted in the center of a dumpling comes out clean. Spoon the warm cobbler onto individual serving plates and serve.

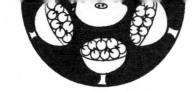

Cherry Cobbler

❖❖

Yield: 6 servings, each with: Calories: 241 • Saturated Fat: 0.69 g • Total Fat: 7.12 g • Cholesterol: 0.22 mg

When mixing up the topping, don't smooth the dough—you want it to be bumpy, and therefore, cobbled.

Fruit

1 (20-ounce) can tart pie cherries in
   juice
½ cup sugar
1 teaspoon almond extract
1 tablespoon instant tapioca

Topping

1 cup all-purpose flour
½ teaspoon cinnamon
1½ teaspoons baking powder
⅓ cup skim milk
3 tablespoons safflower oil
Vanilla ice milk

Preheat the oven to 425° F.

In a medium-size saucepan, combine the cherries (with juice), sugar, almond extract, and tapioca; cook over medium heat until the sugar is dissolved. Pour into a 9-inch pie plate.

For the topping, combine all the topping ingredients in a small mixing bowl, working them into a ball. Drop by spoonfuls over the fruit.

Bake for 25 to 30 minutes. Serve warm with vanilla ice milk, if desired.

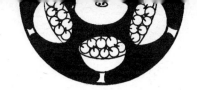

Peach and Berry Bake

❖❖

Yield: 6 servings, each with: Calories: 309 • Saturated Fat: 1.11 g • Total Fat: 10.9 g • Cholesterol: 0.03 mg

Fresh blueberries should look plump and be firm. Rinse them lightly just before you use them; if they become too wet, they will turn to mush.

1 tablespoon cornstarch
1 teaspoon cinnamon
½ teaspoon nutmeg
½ cup sugar
6 ripe peaches, peeled and sliced
1 cup fresh blueberries
½ cup all-purpose flour
½ cup oat flour
1 teaspoon baking powder
¼ cup safflower oil
¼ cup egg substitute (see page 6)
¾ cup orange juice
2 tablespoons lemon juice

Preheat the oven to 375° F.

In a shallow 2-quart baking dish, mix together the cornstarch, cinnamon, nutmeg, and ¼ cup of the sugar. Stir in the peaches and blueberries.

In a small mixing bowl, blend together the flours, baking powder, remaining ¼ cup sugar, and safflower oil. Add the egg substitute and mix well. Distribute the mixture evenly over the fruit. Mix together the orange and lemon juices and pour evenly over the top.

Bake for about 45 minutes; the top should be a golden brown. Serve warm.

89

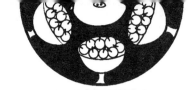

Maple-Glazed Pear Crêpes

Yield: 10 servings, each with: Calories: 110 • Saturated Fat: 0.37 g • Total Fat: 2.88 g • Cholesterol: 0.27 mg

Cinnamon Crêpes

⅔ cup all-purpose flour
⅛ teaspoon cinnamon
⅔ cup skim milk
1 tablespoon safflower oil
3 egg whites

Pear Filling

1 tablespoon tub-style margarine
1 tablespoon light brown sugar
¼ teaspoon cinnamon
⅛ teaspoon salt
4 cups peeled, chopped, firm-ripe pears
1 tablespoon pure maple syrup
1 tablespoon lemon juice
½ teaspoon vanilla extract

In a small bowl, combine the flour and cinnamon; stir well. Gradually add the milk, safflower oil, and egg whites; beat with a wire whisk until smooth. Cover and chill for at least 1 hour.

Lightly grease an 8-inch nonstick skillet with safflower oil and heat over medium heat. Remove from the heat and spoon 2 tablespoons of the crêpe batter into the pan. Quickly tilt the pan in all directions so the batter covers the pan in a thin film. Cook for 2 minutes. Lift the edge of the crêpe and check for doneness. (The crêpe is ready for turning when it can be shaken loose from the pan.) Turn the crêpe over and cook for 1 minute. Place the crêpes on waxed paper. Repeat this process until all the batter is used, stacking the finished crêpes between layers of waxed paper to prevent sticking.

To make the filling, melt the margarine over medium heat in a large skillet; add the brown sugar, cinnamon, and salt and stir well. Add the pears, tossing gently to coat; cook for 10 minutes, stirring occasionally. Add the maple syrup, and cook for 2 minutes more, stirring constantly. Remove from the heat and stir in the lemon juice and vanilla.

To serve, spoon ¼ cup of the filling down the center of each crêpe, and roll up. Serve warm.

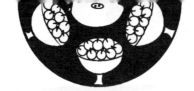

Terri's Special Apple Dumplings

Yield: 12 servings, each with: Calories: 303 • Saturated Fat: 0.43 g • Total Fat: 2.5 g • Cholesterol: 0.35 mg

These dumplings are a lot easier and faster to make than the traditional dumpling. Simply roll them up jelly-roll style, slice, bake, and enjoy!

Dough
¼ cup egg substitute (see page 6)
1 (8-ounce) carton non-fat plain yogurt
2 cups all-purpose flour
2 tablespoons white sugar
2 tablespoons baking powder
¼ teaspoon baking soda
¼ teaspoon salt

Filling
3 baking apples, peeled and coarsely
   chopped
¼ cup white sugar
1½ teaspoon cinnamon
⅛ teaspoon nutmeg

Brown Sugar Sauce
1½ cups water
1¼ cups packed light brown sugar
1 cup white sugar
2 tablespoons cornstarch
2 tablespoons lemon juice
2 tablespoons tub-style margarine

Preheat the oven to 350° F. Grease a 9-inch by 13-inch baking dish with tub-style margarine.

To make the dough, combine the egg substitute and yogurt in a medium-size bowl. Stir in the flour, sugar, baking powder, baking soda, and salt. Mix well.

On a lightly floured surface, roll out the dough to a 12-inch square. Sprinkle the chopped apples evenly on top.

In a small bowl, combine the ¼ cup sugar, cinnamon, and nutmeg; sprinkle evenly over the apples. Very carefully roll up the dough, jelly-roll style. Cut the roll into twelve 1-inch-thick slices. Place the slices, cut side down, in the baking dish.

Stir together the water, brown sugar, 1 cup white sugar, cornstarch, and lemon juice; pour over the dumpling slices. Dot evenly with the margarine.

Bake, uncovered, for 35 to 40 minutes, or until golden. To serve, spoon the warm dumplings into individual dessert dishes.

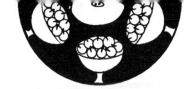

Nectarine Strawberry Puff

Yield: 6 servings, each with: Calories: 179 • Saturated Fat: 0.93 g • Total Fat: 5.97 g • Cholesterol: 1.09 mg

This giant "pancake," has been a long-time favorite of mine.

2 tablespoons tub-style margarine
¾ cup skim milk
¾ cup egg substitute (see page 6)
¾ cup all-purpose flour
¼ teaspoon almond extract
2 cups sliced nectarines
2 cups sliced strawberries
¾ cup non-fat plain yogurt
1 tablespoon honey

Melt the margarine in a 10-inch ovenproof skillet in a 450° F. oven.

Combine the milk and egg substitute with a wire whisk until light and lemon-colored. Beat in the flour and almond extract until smooth.

Remove the skillet from the oven. Pour the batter into the skillet, and return to the oven to bake for 15 minutes, or until the pancake is puffed and browned.

In a small bowl, toss together the nectarines and strawberries. In a separate bowl, mix the yogurt and honey until blended. Serve the hot pancake puff topped with fruit and drizzled with yogurt.

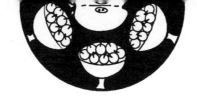

Strawberry-Filled Crêpes

◆◆◆

Yield: 10 servings, each with: Calories: 127 • Saturated Fat: 0.67 g • Total Fat: 2.59 g • Cholesterol: 2.72 mg

A great recipe for entertaining.

Crêpes
1 cup all-purpose flour
1 cup skim milk
½ cup egg substitute (see page 6)
1 tablespoon tub-style margarine,
   melted
⅛ teaspoon almond extract
¼ cup powdered sugar

Strawberry Filling
1 pint non-fat vanilla yogurt
2 tablespoons orange juice
1 pint strawberries, rinsed, hulled,
   and sliced

Stir together the flour, milk, egg substitute, melted margarine, and almond extract. Refrigerate for 30 minutes.

Lightly grease an 8-inch nonstick skillet with safflower oil and heat over medium heat. Spoon about ¼ cup of the batter into the skillet, tilting the pan in all directions. Cook for 1 to 2 minutes, then carefully turn the crêpe over and cook for another 30 seconds. Repeat until all the crêpes are cooked, stacking the finished crêpes between layers of waxed paper.

To make the filling, blend the yogurt with the juice, and stir in the berries.

To serve, spoon ¼ cup of the filling down the center of each crêpe; roll up. Sift powdered sugar lightly over the top.

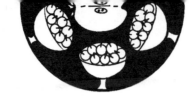

Baked Apples

Yield: 8 servings, each with: Calories: 173 • Saturated Fat: 0.54 g • Total Fat: 4.17 g • Cholesterol: 0 mg

I always make a few extra of these—they're wonderful for breakfast.

¼ cup light brown sugar
1 teaspoon cinnamon
¼ teaspoon nutmeg
1 tablespoon tub-style margarine, melted
⅓ cup raisins
8 medium-size baking apples
¼ cup finely chopped walnuts
1 cup water

Preheat the oven to 375° F.

Combine the sugar, cinnamon, nutmeg, melted margarine, and raisins. Core the apples and pare ⅓ down from the top of each apple. Fill the center of each apple with the sugar mixture, and place it upright in a baking dish. Pour the water around the apples. Bake for 45 to 60 minutes, basting frequently. Serve warm or cold.

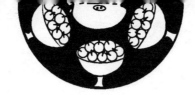

Baked Apples with Apricot Sauce

Yield: 4 servings, each with: Calories: 230 • Saturated Fat: 0.91 g • Total Fat: 9.8 g • Cholesterol: 0 mg

4 baking apples, cored, with a 1-inch strip peeled around the top
½ cup peeled and chopped apricots
½ cup chopped walnuts
¾ cup apricot nectar
2 tablespoons dark brown sugar
¼ teaspoon ground allspice
¼ teaspoon almond extract

Preheat the oven to 350° F.

Place the apples in a baking dish just large enough to hold them. Combine the chopped apricots and walnuts, and fill the center of each apple with the mixture.

In a small saucepan, stir together the apricot nectar, brown sugar, allspice, and almond extract. Bring the mixture to a boil and pour over the apples.

Bake the apples, covered, for 30 minutes. Uncover and bake for another 30 minutes, spooning the nectar over the apples several times while baking. Spoon each apple into a dessert bowl and serve warm.

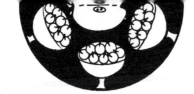

Baked Peaches

◆◆◆

Yield: 4 servings, each with: Calories: 167 • Saturated Fat: 0.58 g • Total Fat: 6.08 g • Cholesterol: 0 mg

Sweet, baked peaches with the tangy addition of orange. If fresh peaches are unavailable, canned peaches can be substituted.

4 medium-ripe peaches, peeled, halved, and pitted
⅓ cup toasted almonds, finely chopped
2 teaspoons orange zest
½ cup powdered sugar
½ cup orange juice

Preheat the oven to 350° F.

Place the peach halves, cut side up, in a 9-inch by 13-inch baking dish. Combine the chopped almonds, the orange zest, and ¼ cup of the powdered sugar. Fill the peach halves with this mixture, dividing it evenly among them. Sprinkle with the orange juice and the remaining ¼ cup powdered sugar.

Bake for 10 minutes and serve warm on individual dessert plates.

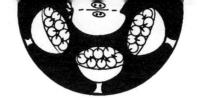

Sherried Pears

❖❖❖

Yield: 6 servings, each with: Calories: 127 • Saturated Fat: 0.35 g • Total Fat: 2.25 g • Cholesterol: 0 mg

A unique recipe: pears sweetened with cream sherry. These are wonderful served as a topping for vanilla ice milk.

6 medium-size pears
⅔ cup packed light brown sugar
½ cup cream sherry
2 tablespoons tub-style margarine
2 tablespoons lemon juice
1 teaspoon cinnamon
½ cup water

Preheat the oven to 350° F.

Halve the pears lengthwise and remove the cores. Place the halves, cut side down, on a cutting board. Make lengthwise cuts from blossom end almost to stem end to fan the pears (be sure not to cut through the stem end). Place the pears, cut side down, in a 6-inch by 10-inch baking dish.

In a small saucepan, combine the brown sugar, sherry, margarine, lemon juice, cinnamon, and water. Cook and stir over medium heat until the mixture is heated through; pour over the pears.

Bake for 35 to 40 minutes, spooning the sauce over the pears occasionally. Serve warm.

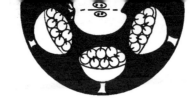

Baked Bananas and Pineapple

❖❖

Yield: 6 servings, each with: Calories: 150 • Saturated Fat: 0.16 g • Total Fat: 0.44 g • Cholesterol: 0 mg

Select bananas that are still a little green; very ripe bananas will cook to mush.

4 bananas, peeled and sliced lengthwise
6 to 8 fresh or canned pineapple slices
2 tablespoons honey
2 tablespoons dark brown sugar
⅛ teaspoon nutmeg

Preheat the oven to 375° F.

Layer the banana and pineapple slices in a small baking dish. Drizzle with the honey; sprinkle with the brown sugar and nutmeg. Bake for 15 minutes. Serve warm.

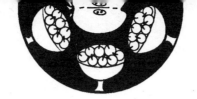

Poached Apples with Banana Cream

Yield: 4 servings, each with: Calories: 175 • Saturated Fat: 0.15 g • Total Fat: 0.67 g • Cholesterol: 0 mg

Tart, baking apples work best for this tasty dessert.

Apples
4 cooking apples
½ cup cranberry juice
2 tablespoons honey
1 (⅛-inch) slice fresh ginger root

Banana Cream
1 egg white
1 tablespoon honey
1 large ripe banana
3 tablespoons lemon juice

Preheat the oven to 375° F.

Core the apples; slice crosswise into thirds, and arrange in a 7-inch by 11-inch baking dish. Combine the cranberry juice, honey, and ginger root; pour over the apples.

Bake for 20 minutes, or until the apples are fork-tender, turning and basting once.

Beat the egg white in a small bowl until it is frothy; gradually add the honey, and beat until well combined. Mash the banana and stir the lemon juice into it. Add to the egg white and beat at high speed until stiff peaks form. This must be prepared and served within 1 hour.

To serve, spoon 3 warm apple slices into each dessert plate and top with the banana cream.

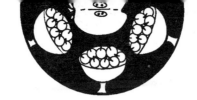

Poached Peaches in Berry Sauce

❖❖

Yield: 4 servings, each with: Calories: 131 • Saturated Fat: 0.40 g • Total Fat: 0.47 g • Cholesterol: 0.35 mg

Juicy, sweet poached peaches flavored with a light raspberry sauce.

1½ cups peach nectar
1 tablespoon orange juice
4 large peaches, peeled and halved
1 pint raspberries
1 teaspoon sugar
¼ cup non-fat plain yogurt

In a medium-size saucepan, bring the peach nectar to a boil and cook for 2 minutes. Stir in the orange juice, then add the peach halves; simmer on low heat for about 5 minutes. Remove from the heat and cool.

Place the raspberries in a blender or food processor and puree. Press through a sieve to remove the seeds.

Stir the sugar into the yogurt.

To serve, pour ¼ cup raspberry puree on each dessert plate. Place 2 chilled peach halves, cut side down, on the sauce and top with a spoonful of sweetened yogurt.

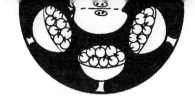

Poached Plums

Yield: 4 servings, each with: Calories: 159 • Saturated Fat: 0.07 g • Total Fat: 0.85 g • Cholesterol: 0 mg

My parents have a beautiful plum tree in their garden. Year after year this old, faithful friend supplies us with an abundance of delicious, juicy fresh plums. This is a new addition to our collection of plum recipes.

⅓ **cup sugar**
½ **cup water**
½ **cup red wine**
1 **tablespoon lemon juice**
2 **whole cloves**
2 **cinnamon sticks**
8 **medium-size plums, quartered**

In a medium-size saucepan, combine the sugar and water. Cook over medium heat until the sugar dissolves, stirring constantly. Stir in the wine, lemon juice, cloves, and cinnamon sticks. Very gently add the plums and bring the mixture to a boil. Reduce the heat to a simmer and continue cooking for 1 to 2 minutes. Take the pan off the burner and remove the cloves and cinnamon sticks with a slotted spoon.

Serve the plums warm, spooning some of the wine mixture over the plums. Top each serving with a dollop of vanilla yogurt, if desired.

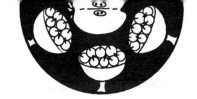

Broiled Apricots

◆◆◆

Yield: 4 servings, each with: Calories: 206 • Saturated Fat: 1.09 g • Total Fat: 6.3 g • Cholesterol: 1.0 mg

The delicious combination of lemon and brown sugar brings out the full flavor of the apricots.

2 tablespoons tub-style margarine, melted
1 tablespoon lemon juice
1 pound firm-ripe apricots, halved (do not peel)
⅓ cup packed dark brown sugar
⅛ teaspoon nutmeg
1 (8-ounce) carton non-fat plain yogurt

Grease an 8-inch by 12-inch baking dish with safflower oil.

In a small bowl, combine the melted margarine and lemon juice. Arrange the apricot halves, cut side up, in a single layer in the baking dish, and drizzle the fruit with the lemon-margarine mixture. Sprinkle the brown sugar evenly over the apricots.

Broil about 6 inches below the heat for 3 to 5 minutes, or until the brown sugar is dissolved and the topping is bubbling.

Stir the freshly grated nutmeg into the yogurt.

Serve the fruit hot with a dollop of yogurt spooned over the top.

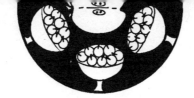

Broiled Pineapple Slices

Yield: 4 servings, each with: Calories: 55 • Saturated Fat: 0.01 g • Total Fat: 0.08 g • Cholesterol: 0 mg

The pineapple is the symbol of hospitality. Choose the ripest pineapple you can find for this recipe; just check for tenderness and smell for sweetness. Canned pineapple slices, packed in their own juice, are equally delicious.

½ teaspoon grated orange zest
½ cup orange juice
2 tablespoons dark brown sugar
8 pineapple slices

In a small mixing bowl, blend together the orange zest, orange juice, and brown sugar.

Place the pineapple slices on an unheated broiler rack in a broiler pan. Using a pastry brush, generously brush on the orange juice mixture. Broil 3 to 4 inches from the heat for about 4 to 5 minutes, or until heated through, brushing occasionally with the orange juice mixture. Remove the slices from the broiler pan with a spatula and serve immediately.

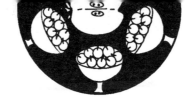

Sautéed Apple Wedges

❖❖

Yield: 6 servings, each with: Calories: 249 • Saturated Fat: 1.38 g • Total Fat: 8.05 g • Cholesterol: 0 mg

¼ cup tub-style margarine
6 apples, each cut into 8 wedges and
   seeded
1 cup apple brandy
2 tablespoons light brown sugar
¼ teaspoon ground cloves
½ teaspoon ground ginger

In a medium-size skillet, melt the margarine over medium heat. Add the apples and sauté until just tender, about 4 minutes. Stir in the apple brandy, sugar, cloves, and ginger. Stirring gently and constantly, cook over low heat for 3 minutes. Remove the apples to a serving dish. Increase the heat to high and boil the liquid to reduce by half. Pour the sauce over the apples and serve.

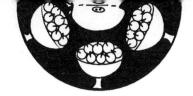

Brandied Applesauce

Yield: 5 servings, each with: Calories: 160 • Saturated Fat: 0.92 g • Total Fat: 0.57 g • Cholesterol: 0 mg

Apples and brandy—as perfect a match as you can get. This rich applesauce is a unique and welcome change from the traditional.

**2 pounds cooking apples, peeled and
   coarsely chopped**
½ cup water
3 tablespoons light brown sugar
¼ cup brandy

In a 3-quart saucepan, stir together the apples, water, and brown sugar. Bring this to a boil; reduce the heat to simmer and continue cooking for another 20 minutes, stirring often.

Mash the apples with a potato masher. You may need to add a little more water at this point to keep the apples from sticking to the pan. Blend in the brandy and cover. Cook on low heat for 5 minutes longer. The flavor of the sauce is at its fullest when still warm. Serve with a plateful of Rolled Oat Cookies (page 146).

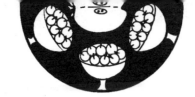

Cranberry Applesauce

❖❖

Yield: 8 servings, each with: Calories: 199 • Saturated Fat: 0.11 g • Total Fat: 0.67 g • Cholesterol: 0 mg

A colorful, sweet-tart variation of an old favorite.

6 large cooking apples, peeled and cut into quarters
⅔ cup water
2 cups whole-berry cranberry sauce

Place the apples and water in a medium-size saucepan; heat to boiling over high heat. Reduce the heat to low and simmer, uncovered, until tender, about 10 to 15 minutes. Stir in the cranberry sauce and heat through. Serve warm or cold.

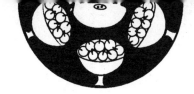

Minted Peach Raspberry Compote

Yield: 4 servings, each with: Calories: 116 • Saturated Fat: 0.02 g • Total Fat: 0.33 g • Cholesterol: 0 mg

Serve this colorful fruit combination in champagne glasses—it'll make your whole meal seem special.

⅓ **cup water**
⅓ **cup sugar**
1 to 2 **tablespoons lemon juice**
2 **tablespoons chopped fresh mint leaves**
3 **medium-size ripe peaches, peeled and sliced**
1½ **cups raspberries, rinsed and drained**

In a medium-size saucepan, combine the water and sugar. Bring to a boil over high heat; boil for 30 seconds, stirring until the sugar dissolves. Remove from the heat; stir in the lemon juice and chopped mint. Refrigerate until cold.

Lightly mix the peaches and raspberries with the cooled mint sauce. Serve at once, or cover and refrigerate for up to 3 hours.

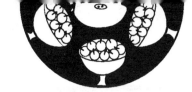

Caramel Oranges

❖•❖

Yield: 4 servings, each with: Calories: 219 • Saturated Fat: 0.99 g • Total Fat: 5.85 g • Cholesterol: 0 mg

½ cup packed light brown sugar
2 tablespoons tub-style margarine
¼ teaspoon grated orange zest
1 cinnamon stick
4 navel oranges, peeled and sliced into
   rounds

In a medium-heavy saucepan, combine the brown sugar, margarine, orange zest, and cinnamon stick and cook for about 3 minutes, stirring frequently. The mixture should have a syrupy consistency. Remove the cinnamon stick.

To serve, place overlapping orange rounds on 4 individual dessert plates. Drizzle the caramel sauce over the orange slices and serve at once.

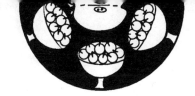

Melon Mélange

◆◆

Yield: 4 servings, each with: Calories: 80 • Saturated Fat: 0.08 g • Total Fat: 0.48 g • Cholesterol: 0 mg

Simple pleasures are the best, and this quick-to-prepare summer fruit dessert is no exception. Scrumptious when served with warm Oatmeal Cookies (page 133).

1 cup seeded watermelon balls
1 cup honeydew melon balls
1 cup cantaloupe melon balls
1 cup diced green apple (do not peel)
1 teaspoon grated orange zest
¾ cup apple juice
Fresh mint

Combine the fruit, orange zest, and apple juice in a large bowl. Toss to blend well; cover and chill. Serve in fruit cups or stemmed glasses with a sprig of mint.

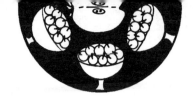

Grape White Wine Dessert

Yield: 4 servings, each with: Calories: 146 • Saturated Fat: 0.14 g • Total Fat: 0.43 g • Cholesterol: 0.25 mg

Be sure to chill the gelatin until it begins to thicken or the grapes will all settle to the bottom of the glass when they are added.

⅓ cup sugar
⅛ teaspoon salt
1 tablespoon plain gelatin
⅓ cup lemon juice
1 cup boiling water
½ cup white wine
¾ cup halved seedless green grapes
¾ cup halved seedless red grapes
4 tablespoons non-fat plain yogurt

In a small mixing bowl, blend the sugar, salt, and gelatin. Stir in the lemon juice and set aside for 5 minutes to soften.

Add the boiling water. Stir until the gelatin and sugar dissolve; add the wine. Chill this mixture until it begins to thicken; add the grapes and mix well.

Spoon the mixture into 4 dessert glasses. Chill until set.

To serve, top each glass with a tablespoon of non-fat yogurt.

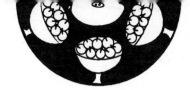

Cinnamon Grapes

❖❖

Yield: 4 servings, each with: Calories: 138 • Saturated Fat: 0.53 g • Total Fat: 1.28 g • Cholesterol: 1.42 mg

½ cup non-fat vanilla yogurt
¼ teaspoon cinnamon
2 cups seedless green grapes
2 cups seedless red grapes

Combine the vanilla yogurt and the cinnamon in a bowl; blend well. Add the grapes and toss until they're evenly coated. Cover and chill until serving time.

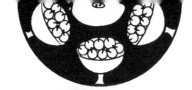

Blueberry Nectarine Toss

❖❖❖

Yield: 4 servings, each with: Calories: 136 • Saturated Fat: 0.11 g • Total Fat: 0.76 g • Cholesterol: 0 mg

Here is a good way to take advantage of the bountiful summer fruits. By serving them as simply as possible, you can really appreciate their true flavors.

4 nectarines, peeled and sliced in
   wedges
½ pint fresh blueberries
3 tablespoons honey
¼ teaspoon grated orange zest

In a large bowl, toss together the nectarines, blueberries, honey, and orange zest. Spoon into dessert glasses.

Note: A quick way to peel nectarines is to drop them into boiling water for 10 seconds. Remove them from the water and let them cool enough to handle. Then use a small knife to remove the skins—they will slip off easily.

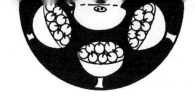

Plum Crème

◆◆◆

Yield: 4 servings, each with: Calories: 138 • Saturated Fat: 0.1 g • Total Fat: 0.51 g • Cholesterol: 1.0 mg

Italian plums give a tart flavor and a brilliant deep color to this simple and elegant dessert.

4 plums, sliced
1 cup non-fat plain yogurt
½ teaspoon vanilla extract
½ teaspoon almond extract
¼ cup honey
1 tablespoon plain gelatin
2 tablespoons water

In a blender, combine the plums, yogurt, and vanilla and almond extracts. Blend until smooth; add the honey.

Combine the gelatin and water in small saucepan. Stir over low heat until dissolved. Add to the plum mixture in the blender, and process for about 10 seconds.

Spoon into dessert glasses and chill until set.

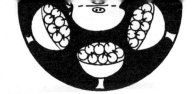

Rhubarb Honey Sauce

Yield: 6 servings, each with: Calories: 60 • Saturated Fat: 0.01 g • Total Fat: 0.16 g • Cholesterol: 0 mg

This is delicious served warm over banana slices, or try serving it chilled over vanilla ice milk.

4 cups rhubarb, cut into 1-inch slices
4 tablespoons honey
1 to 2 tablespoons water
⅛ teaspoon cinnamon
¼ teaspoon grated orange zest

In a medium-size saucepan, combine the rhubarb, honey, water, and cinnamon. Cover and simmer over a low heat for about 10 minutes, or until the fruit is tender. Stir in the orange zest. Serve warm or chilled.

5
Puddings and Mousses

Puddings are often thought of as old-fashioned. But they have endured as a favorite dessert because of their versatility and because of their flavor and texture. Mousses are usually looked upon as elegant and sophisticated. Puddings are creamy and heavy because they are stirred and baked and usually thickened by a starch, whereas mousses are lighter because they are whipped, either with egg whites or milk products. Choose the one that best complements your mood, from the traditional Rice Pudding to the richer taste of Mocha Mousse.

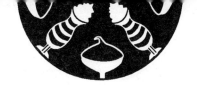

Brown Rice Pudding

Yield: 8 servings, each with: Calories: 188 • Saturated Fat: 0.35 g • Total Fat: 1.87 g • Cholesterol: 1.57 mg

The quintessential pudding. The brown rice makes it very flavorful and hearty.

2 cups cooked brown rice
3 cups skim milk
¼ cup light brown sugar
1 cup raisins
~~¼ teaspoon nutmeg~~
¼ teaspoon cinnamon
¾ cup egg substitute (see page 6)

Preheat the oven to 325° F.

Combine all of the ingredients in a large bowl and mix well. Pour the mixture into a greased 2-quart casserole, and bake for about 1 hour, or until set. This is delicious served either hot or cold.

[handwritten annotations:]

¼ + 2T sugar
½ C raisins
1 3/4 t cinnamon
2 Jumbo eggs
bake in white oblong pyrex pan.

4/14/17
Good recipe!

1st time
uncovered (?) till half done, then cover?

2nd time
cover at first 30 min
uncovered 30 min + 8 min
+ covered 8½ min + 5 min cvrd 250°

119

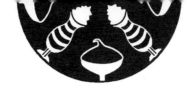

Raisin Rice Pudding

❖❖

Yield: 6 servings, each with: Calories: 136 • Saturated Fat: 0.23 g • Total Fat: 1.3 g • Cholesterol: 1.06 mg

Try serving this topped with either Blueberry Sauce (page 169) or Strawberry Sauce (page 168).

1 cup cooked white rice
2 tablespoons sugar
½ teaspoon cinnamon
1½ cups skim milk
½ cup egg substitute (see page 6)
1 teaspoon vanilla extract
½ cup raisins
Freshly ground nutmeg

Preheat the oven to 350° F.

In a large bowl, combine the cooked rice, sugar, and cinnamon. Stir in the milk, the egg substitute, and the vanilla; add the raisins and mix well.

Pour into a lightly greased 1-quart baking dish. Sprinkle the nutmeg over the top. Bake the pudding for 1 hour, or until a knife inserted at the center comes out clean. Serve warm or cold.

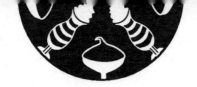

Orange Rice Custard

❖❖

Yield: 4 servings, each with: Calories: 157 • Saturated Fat: 0.19 g • Total Fat: 1.05 g • Cholesterol: 1.3 mg

1¼ cups skim milk
¼ cup sugar
¼ cup egg substitute (see page 6)
¾ cup cooked white rice
1 teaspoon grated orange zest
½ teaspoon vanilla extract
2 teaspoons sugar
1 orange, cut into wedges

Preheat the oven to 350° F.

In a medium-size saucepan, scald the milk and stir in the ¼ cup sugar. Slowly add the egg substitute, stirring constantly. Stir in the cooked rice, ½ teaspoon of the orange zest, and the vanilla. Pour the mixture into four 6-ounce custard cups. Set the cups in a shallow baking pan that has 1 inch of hot water on the bottom.

Bake for 30 minutes, or until a knife inserted in the center of a custard cup comes out clean.

Blend together the remaining ½ teaspoon orange zest and the 2 teaspoons of sugar. Sprinkle this mixture over the tops of the hot custard. Cool. Serve the cooled pudding topped with orange wedges.

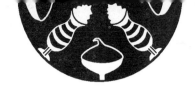

Tapioca Pudding

Yield: 6 servings, each with: Calories: 99 • Saturated Fat: 0.1 g • Total Fat: 0.15 g • Cholesterol: 1.33 mg

A delicious old standby that can be served warm or cold. My favorite way of serving it is chilled, topped with Creamy Whipped Topping (page 6) and a sprinkle of freshly grated nutmeg.

2 cups skim milk
4 tablespoons instant tapioca
⅓ cup sugar
1 teaspoon vanilla extract
2 egg whites

In a medium-size saucepan, combine the milk, tapioca, and half of the sugar; let stand for 5 minutes. Then cook over medium heat, stirring constantly until it comes to a boil. Remove from the heat; add the vanilla. Let the mixture cool for 30 minutes.

Beat the egg whites until foamy, then slowly add the remaining sugar while continuing to beat at medium speed until soft peaks form. Fold this into the cooled tapioca.

Spoon into 6 individual dessert glasses, and chill before serving.

Almond Peach Tapioca

❖❖

Yield: 6 servings, each with: Calories: 100 • Saturated Fat: 0.1 g • Total Fat: 0.18 g • Cholesterol: 1.33 mg

A delicious creamy pudding that can also be made with nectarines or apricots.

2 cups skim milk
4 tablespoons instant tapioca
4 tablespoons sugar
½ teaspoon almond extract
2 egg whites
1 cup peeled and diced peaches

In a medium-size saucepan, combine the milk, tapioca, and 2 tablespoons of the sugar; let stand for 5 minutes. Then cook over medium heat, stirring constantly until it comes to a boil. Remove from the heat, add the almond extract, and allow to cool for 30 minutes.

Beat the egg whites until foamy; slowly add the remaining 2 tablespoons sugar while continuing to beat at medium speed until soft peaks form.

Stir the diced peaches into the cooked mixture. Gently fold in the egg whites, blending well.

Spoon into 6 individual dessert glasses and chill before serving.

Apricot Pudding

Yield: 8 servings, each with: Calories: 247 • Saturated Fat: 0.54 g • Total Fat: 3.09 g • Cholesterol: 0.25 mg

Pudding

1 cup all-purpose flour
⅔ cup packed light brown sugar
1½ teaspoons baking powder
½ cup skim milk
¼ teaspoon vanilla extract

Apricot Sauce

1 cup finely chopped dried apricots
2 cups water
⅔ cups packed light brown sugar
2 tablespoons tub-style margarine
¼ teaspoon cinnamon
¼ teaspoon allspice

In a medium-size mixing bowl, stir together the flour, brown sugar, and baking powder. Add the milk and vanilla; stir until uniformly moistened. Spread the batter evenly in a 9-inch square baking dish.

In a medium-size saucepan, combine all the sauce ingredients and bring them to a boil over high heat. Reduce the heat to medium, and cook for 2 to 3 minutes longer, stirring often.

Pour the apricot sauce over the batter, and bake for 35 minutes, or until the cake layer that forms on top is firm to the touch and nicely browned.

To serve, spoon the warm pudding into individual dessert bowls and top with a dollop of Creamy Whipped Topping (page 6), if desired.

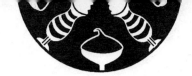

Pineapple Cheese Pudding

❖❖❖

Yield: 6 servings, each with: Calories: 158 • Saturated Fat: 0.91 g • Total Fat: 3.74 g • Cholesterol: 3.4 mg

2 cups low-fat cottage cheese
½ cup egg substitute (see page 6)
1 tablespoon tub-style margarine, melted
½ teaspoon vanilla extract
⅓ cup sugar
2 tablespoons all-purpose flour
1 (8-ounce) can unsweetened crushed pineapple, drained
⅛ teaspoon cinnamon

Preheat the oven to 425° F. Lightly grease a 2-quart baking dish with safflower oil.

Combine the cottage cheese, egg substitute, margarine, and vanilla in a blender. Blend on high speed for 10 seconds. Add the sugar, flour, and pineapple; blend an additional 10 seconds.

Pour the mixture into the prepared baking dish and sprinkle with the cinnamon. Place this dish in a larger pan; fill the large pan with an inch of water. Bake for 10 minutes; reduce the heat to 350° F., and bake for 40 minutes longer, or until a knife inserted into the center of the pudding comes out clean. I like to serve this while it's still warm.

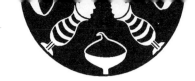

Flan

❖❖❖

Yield: 6 servings, each with: Calories: 147 • Saturated Fat: 0.27 g • Total Fat: 1.71 g • Cholesterol: 1.87 mg

Flan is a traditional Mexican custard that is rich and sweet. We serve this at our house when we have Mexican food for dinner.

6 tablespoons sugar
¾ cup egg substitute (see page 6)
⅓ cup sugar
2⅔ cups skim milk, scalded
¾ teaspoon vanilla extract

Preheat the oven to 350° F.

Melt the 6 tablespoons sugar over medium heat until golden brown, stirring constantly; pour at once into six 6-ounce custard cups. Tilt the cups to coat evenly.

In a medium-size saucepan, combine the egg substitute and ⅓ cup sugar. Stir in the scalded milk and vanilla; heat through. Carefully pour the liquid into the custard cups. Set the cups in a shallow baking pan filled with 1 inch of water.

Bake for 25 to 30 minutes, or until a knife inserted in the center comes out clean; cool to room temperature. Then chill for 2 hours, or until firm.

To serve, loosen the edges with a knife and invert the cups onto dessert plates.

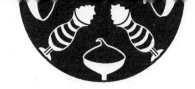

Mocha Mousse

❖❖❖

Yield: 8 servings, each with: Calories: 83 • Saturated Fat: 0.38 g • Total Fat: 0.62 g • Cholesterol: 1.0 mg

This is one of the lightest and richest mousses I know. For a special touch, garnish with fresh berries.

¼ cup unsweetened cocoa powder
¼ cup sugar
¼ cup cornstarch
1 teaspoon instant espresso coffee
   powder
2 cups skim milk
1½ teaspoons vanilla extract
4 egg whites
¼ teaspoon cream of tartar
2 tablespoons sugar

In a 2-quart saucepan, combine the cocoa, ¼ cup sugar, cornstarch, and the coffee powder. Gradually stir in the milk until blended and smooth. Cook over medium heat for about 5 minutes, stirring constantly, until the mixture boils gently and is thick enough to coat the back of a metal spoon. Remove from the heat; stir in the vanilla. Pour into a large bowl; cover and refrigerate until cold, about 45 minutes.

Beat the egg whites and cream of tartar until foamy; beat in the remaining 2 tablespoons of sugar gradually until stiff peaks form. Fold the egg whites into the mocha mixture and blend thoroughly.

Spoon into 8 dessert glasses and chill for at least 1 hour before serving.

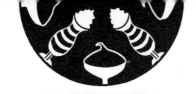

Raspberry Mousse

❖❖

Yield: 6 servings, each with: Calories: 111 • Saturated Fat: 0.03 g • Total Fat: 0.26 g • Cholesterol: 0.67 mg

This dessert requires a little extra effort, but it's always worth the time—it gets rave reviews.

2 cups fresh raspberries
⅓ cup water
1 envelope unflavored gelatin
3 tablespoons water
½ cup sugar
½ teaspoon grated lemon zest
1 tablespoon fresh lemon juice
⅓ cup instant non-fat dry milk
3 egg whites

Gently rinse the raspberries; drain. In a blender, process the raspberries until smooth. Strain the mixture and discard the seeds.

Place the ⅓ cup water in a small glass bowl and place in the freezer for about 25 minutes.

Sprinkle the gelatin over the remaining 3 tablespoons of water in a small saucepan; let stand for 1 minute. Then cook over low heat until the gelatin dissolves, stirring constantly. Remove from the heat. Add ¼ cup of the sugar, the lemon zest, and the lemon juice, stirring until the sugar dissolves. Blend with the raspberry puree. Cover and chill for 25 minutes, or until slightly thickened, stirring frequently. Set aside.

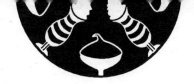

In a small mixing bowl, add the instant milk to the partially frozen water; beat at high speed for 5 minutes. Set aside.

In a large mixing bowl, beat the egg whites at medium speed until soft peaks form. Add the remaining ¼ cup of sugar gradually, beating until soft peaks form. Gently stir the egg white mixture into the raspberry mixture. Carefully fold the milk mixture into the raspberry mixture.

Spoon into 6 dessert dishes and chill for at least 3 hours before serving.

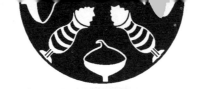

Citrus Mousse with Fresh Fruit

✦✦✦

Yield: 6 servings, each with: Calories: 98 • Saturated Fat: 0.1 g • Total Fat: 0.33 g • Cholesterol: 1.33 mg

A light and refreshing summer dessert. The nutritional analysis for this recipe is based on using 2 cups of sliced fresh strawberries as the garnish for the mousse.

1 cup skim milk
1 tablespoon gelatin
¼ cup honey
1 teaspoon grated orange zest
1 cup non-fat plain yogurt
2 cups sliced fresh fruit, a combination
   of your choice
Mint leaves

Stir the milk into the gelatin in a medium-size saucepan; let stand for 5 minutes. Cook over medium heat until the gelatin is dissolved, stirring constantly. Remove from the heat.

Stir in the honey and the orange zest. When cooled slightly, blend in the non-fat yogurt until it is smooth. Pour the mixture into 6 custard cups. Cover each and chill in the refrigerator for about 3 hours, or until set.

To serve, unmold the mousse onto 6 individual dessert plates. Spoon the sliced fresh fruit over the top and garnish with mint leaves.

6
Cookies

Freshly baked cookies add a touch of home-made goodness to every occasion. From the most casual family fare to the finishing touch for any dinner party, a plateful of warm, fragrant cookies are always welcome. Cookies are synonymous with so many happy times: welcoming new neighbors to the neighborhood, children's class parties, holiday gift giving, a simple personal thank-you gift for a dear friend.

When baking cookies, choose your pans carefully. Heavy-gauge aluminum, slightly smaller than the inside of your oven (so the heat can circulate evenly) is usually the best. The cookie sheets that I use are heavy-gauge, measuring $16\frac{1}{2}$ inches by $12\frac{1}{2}$ inches.

As for greasing the pans, it comes down to a matter of preference. I rarely grease my pans anymore. Many baking sheets are coated with a nonstick surface now, and most cookies have enough shortening to prevent sticking. If greasing of the pan is required, I always season lightly with tub-style margarine. As an alternative to greasing, you can line your baking sheets with parchment or waxed paper.

Be sure to allow plenty of room on the baking sheet for cookies to spread out while baking. Allow time for the sheet to cool before wiping it clean, regreasing it if needed, and baking another tray.

It's important to use the right size pan when baking bar cookies. If the pan is larger than recommended, the dough will be thin and the bars will become dry from overbaking. If the pan is too small, the dough will be too thick and will not bake completely.

Preheat your oven for at least 15 minutes before baking. Cool the cookies on wire racks before storing.

The nutritional analysis provided for each recipe is based on a single cookie. How many cookies you will eat is up to you!

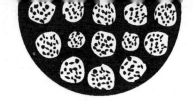

Oatmeal Cookies

❖❖❖

Yield: 48 cookies, each with: Calories: 99 • Saturated Fat: 0.85 g • Total Fat: 5.77 g • Cholesterol: 0.01 mg

1 cup tub-style margarine, at room
    temperature
1 cup packed light brown sugar
½ cup egg substitute (see page 6)
1 teaspoon cinnamon
1 teaspoon vanilla extract
2 cups rolled oats
1 cup chopped nuts (walnuts or pecans)
1 cup whole wheat flour
1 cup all-purpose flour
½ teaspoon baking soda
½ teaspoon baking powder
½ teaspoon salt

Preheat the oven to 375° F. Grease 2 baking sheets or line with parchment or waxed paper.

In a large mixing bowl, combine the margarine, brown sugar, and egg substitute; beat for 2 minutes at medium speed. Add the remaining ingredients; blend on low speed until thoroughly mixed. Drop by teaspoonfuls, 2 inches apart, onto the baking sheets. Bake for 10 minutes, or until slightly browned. Allow the cookies to sit on the baking sheet for 2 to 3 minutes before removing then to a wire rack to finish cooling.

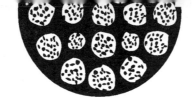

Zucchini Oat Cookies

Yield: 60 cookies, each with: Calories: 54 • Saturated Fat: 0.3 g • Total Fat: 1.75 g • Cholesterol: 0 mg

½ cup tub-style margarine, at room temperature
¾ cup honey
¼ cup egg substitute (see page 6)
2 cups whole wheat flour
1 teaspoon baking soda
¼ teaspoon salt
1 teaspoon cinnamon
¼ teaspoon allspice
1 cup grated zucchini
1 cup rolled oats
1 cup chopped dates

Preheat the oven to 375° F. Grease 2 baking sheets with tub-style margarine or spray with a vegetable oil.

In a large mixing bowl, blend together the margarine, honey, and egg substitute; beat well.

Sift together the flour, baking soda, salt, cinnamon, and allspice. Add the flour mixture alternately with the grated zucchini to the beaten egg mixture. Stir in the rolled oats and the dates.

Drop by the teaspoonful 2 inches apart onto the baking sheets. Bake for 10 to 12 minutes. Immediately remove the cookies from the baking sheets to cool on wire racks.

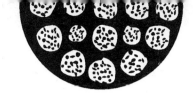

Raisin Applesauce Cookies

◆◆

Yield: 36 cookies, each with: Calories: 106 • Saturated Fat: 0.6 g • Total Fat: 3.95 g • Cholesterol: 0 mg

These cookies are hearty, spicy, and perfect for packed lunches.

½ cup tub-style margarine, at room temperature
½ cup dark brown sugar
½ cup white sugar
1 cup unsweetened applesauce
2 cups all-purpose flour
1 teaspoon cinnamon
½ teaspoon freshly grated nutmeg
1 teaspoon baking soda
2 teaspoons baking powder
2 cups rolled oats
½ cup raisins
½ cup chopped walnuts

Preheat the oven to 375° F. Grease 2 baking sheets with tub-style margarine or spray with vegetable oil.

In a large mixing bowl, cream the margarine and the sugars until light and fluffy; add the applesauce. Sift together the flour, cinnamon, nutmeg, baking soda, and baking powder; add to the applesauce mixture. Stir in the rolled oats, raisins, and chopped nuts.

Drop by the tablespoonful 2 inches apart onto the cookie sheets; bake for 10 to 12 minutes. Allow the cookies to set on the baking sheets for about 3 minutes before removing to wire racks to cool completely.

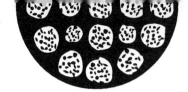

Pecan Orange Cookies

❖❖❖

Yield: 36 cookies, each with: Calories: 62 • Saturated Fat: 0.58 g • Total Fat: 4.34 g • Cholesterol: 0.01 mg

These are delicate, tea-type cookies.

½ cup tub-style margarine
⅓ cup sugar
¼ cup egg substitute (see page 6)
2 tablespoons orange juice
1 cup all-purpose flour
½ teaspoon salt
½ teaspoon grated orange zest
¾ cup chopped pecans
About ½ cup powdered sugar

Preheat the oven to 350° F.

In a large mixing bowl, cream the margarine and sugar. Blend in the egg substitute and the orange juice. Add the flour, salt, and orange zest; mix well. Stir in the chopped pecans.

Drop by rounded teaspoonfuls onto ungreased baking sheets, and bake for 9 to 12 minutes. While still hot, roll in powdered sugar. Cool on wire racks.

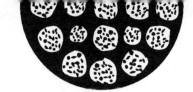

Butter Pecan Balls

Yield: 48 cookies, each with: Calories: 89 • Saturated Fat: 0.93 g • Total Fat: 7.21 g • Cholesterol: 0 mg

Sometimes referred to as Mexican Wedding Cakes, Butter Pecan Balls are a light-textured cookie with a buttery taste.

1 cup tub-style margarine, at room temperature
⅓ cup granulated sugar
2 teaspoons vanilla extract
2 cups cake flour
Dash salt
2 cups finely chopped pecans
¼ cup powdered sugar

Preheat the oven to 325° F.

In a large mixing bowl, cream the margarine and granulated sugar. Add the vanilla, cake flour, salt, and nuts; blend thoroughly. The dough will be stiff. Shape the dough into 1-inch balls.

Bake on an ungreased cookie sheet for about 20 minutes, or until the cookies are set; do not brown. Cool the cookies slightly, then roll them in the powdered sugar. Store in a covered container, separating the layers with waxed paper.

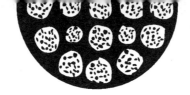

Brian's Peanut Butter Cookies

❖❖

Yield: 30 cookies, each with: Calories: 95 • Saturated Fat: 0.69 g • Total Fat: 3.82 g • Cholesterol: 0.01 mg

Whole wheat flour can be substituted for the all-purpose flour. These are soft cookies, and the flavor gets even better after a day or two in the cookie jar.

¼ **cup tub-style margarine, at room temperature**
½ **cup unsweetened smooth or chunky peanut butter**
½ **cup packed light brown sugar**
½ **cup honey**
¼ **cup egg substitute (see page 6)**
1¼ **cups all-purpose flour**
½ **teaspoon baking powder**
¼ **teaspoon salt**
½ **teaspoon baking soda**
¼ **cup white sugar**

Preheat the oven to 375° F. Grease 2 baking sheets with tub-style margarine or spray with vegetable oil.

In a large mixing bowl, combine the margarine, peanut butter, brown sugar, honey, and egg substitute; mix well. Add the dry ingredients (except for the white sugar), and blend thoroughly. Chill for 1 hour.

Shape the dough into 1-inch balls and roll in the white sugar. Place the balls 3 inches apart on the cookie sheets. Take a fork, dip the tines first into water and then into the white sugar; then press the cookie down with the back of the fork in a crisscross fashion. Bake for 10 to 12 minutes. Remove from the pans immediately and cool on wire racks.

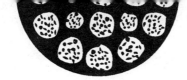

Molasses Crinkles

Yield: 36 cookies , each with: Calories: 94 • Saturated Fat: 0.67 g • Total Fat: 3.98 g • Cholesterol: 0.01 mg

Similar to snickerdoodles, these cookies are much more flavorful and spicy.

2¼ cups all-purpose flour
1 teaspoon baking soda
½ teaspoon salt
1 teaspoon cinnamon
1 teaspoon ground ginger
½ teaspoon ground nutmeg
½ teaspoon cloves
1 cup packed light brown sugar
¾ cup tub-style margarine, at room
    temperature
¼ cup unsulphured molasses
¼ cup egg substitute (see page 6)
¼ cup white sugar

Preheat the oven to 375° F.

In a large mixing bowl, combine the flour, baking soda, salt, cinnamon, ginger, nutmeg, and cloves; set aside.

Beat together the brown sugar, margarine, molasses, and egg substitute until well blended. Stir in the flour mixture. Cover and refrigerate for 1 hour.

Shape the dough into 1-inch balls and roll them in the sugar. Place the balls on ungreased cookie sheets, 3 inches apart. Bake for 10 to 12 minutes, or until the tops have cracked. Remove from the pans immediately and cool on wire racks.

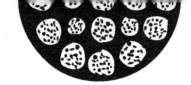

Cocoa Softies

❖❖

Yield: 30 cookies, each with: Calories: 32 • Saturated Fat: 0.1 g • Total Fat: 0. 38 g • Cholesterol: 0.01 mg

These cookies are soft, slightly chewy, and incredibly delicious!

⅓ cup sugar
¼ cup unsweetened cocoa powder
½ cup egg substitute (see page 6)
¾ cup all-purpose flour
¼ teaspoon baking powder
¼ teaspoon cinnamon
¼ teaspoon salt
¼ cup water
1 teaspoon vanilla extract
¼ teaspoon lemon extract
3 egg whites
¼ teaspoon cream of tartar
¼ cup sugar

Preheat the oven to 350° F. Grease 2 baking sheets with tub-style margarine and lightly dust with flour.

In a small bowl, blend together the ⅓ cup sugar, the cocoa, and the egg substitute; beat until very thick. Mix in the flour, baking powder, cinnamon, and salt. Add the water, and the extracts.

In a large mixing bowl, beat the egg whites and the cream of tartar. Slowly add the remaining ¼ cup sugar; beat until it looks stiff and shiny. Fold the egg and flour mixture into the egg whites.

Drop by full teaspoonfuls, at least 2 inches apart, onto the prepared baking sheets. Bake for 10 to 12 minutes. Remove from the oven and cool on wire racks.

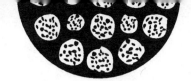

Chocolate Nut Cookies

Yield: 30 cookies, each with: Calories: 80 • Saturated Fat: 0.46 g • Total Fat: 3.08 g • Cholesterol: 0.07 mg

These have a fudge-like flavor and are very easy to prepare.

¼ cup tub-style margarine, at room temperature
1 cup sugar
1¾ cups all-purpose flour
¼ cup unsweetened cocoa powder
1 teaspoon baking soda
¼ teaspoon cinnamon
⅛ teaspoon salt
½ cup skim milk
½ cup chopped pecans

Preheat the oven to 350° F. Grease 2 baking sheets with tub-style margarine or spray with vegetable oil.

In a large mixing bowl, cream the margarine and sugar together until light and fluffy. Add the flour, cocoa, soda, cinnamon, and salt; blend well. Add the milk and pecans, mixing until thoroughly blended.

Drop by the tablespoonful 2 inches apart onto the baking sheets; bake for 10 to 12 minutes. Remove from the baking sheets immediately to cool on wire racks. If desired, frost the cooled cookies with Chocolate Buttercream Icing (page 170).

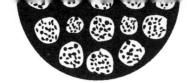

Favorite Sugar Cookies

Yield: 36 cookies, each with: Calories: 74 • Saturated Fat: 0.46 • Total Fat: 2.7 g • Cholesterol: 0.02 mg

When I was a child, this was one of my very favorite cookies. The hint of lemon inside the cookie and the sprinkle of freshly grated nutmeg on top are the magical ingredients.

½ **cup tub-style margarine, at room temperature**
¼ **teaspoon salt**
1 **tablespoon lemon zest**
1 **cup sugar**
½ **teaspoon lemon extract**
¼ **cup egg substitute (see page 6)**
2 **tablespoons skim milk**
2 **cups all-purpose flour**
1 **teaspoon baking powder**
½ **teaspoon baking soda**
Freshly grated nutmeg
¼ **cup sugar**

Preheat the oven to 400° F. Grease 2 baking sheets.

Cream together the margarine, salt, lemon zest, 1 cup sugar, and lemon extract. Blend in the egg substitute, milk, and flour. Stir in the baking powder and baking soda.

Drop by the rounded teaspoonful 2 inches apart onto the cookie sheets. To flatten each cookie, grease the bottom of a drinking glass and dip in the ¼ cup sugar; press each cookie to a thickness of about ¼ inch. (Re-dip the glass in sugar after pressing each cookie.) Sprinkle the nutmeg on the cookies. Bake for 8 to 10 minutes; the edges of the cookies will start to brown. Immediately remove from the cookie sheets to cool on wire racks.

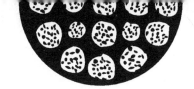

Ginger Creams

Yield: 48 cookies, each with: Calories: 69 • Saturated Fat: 0.4 g • Total Fat: 2.35 g • Cholesterol: 0.01 mg

The flavor of these cake-like cookies gets even better after a day or so—if they last!

½ cup sugar
⅓ cup tub-style margarine, at room
    temperature
¼ cup egg substitute (see page 6)
½ cup light molasses
½ cup warm water
1 teaspoon ground ginger
½ teaspoon salt
½ teaspoon baking soda
½ teaspoon nutmeg
½ teaspoon cloves
½ teaspoon cinnamon
2 cups all-purpose flour
Buttercream Icing (page 170)

Preheat the oven to 400° F.

In a large mixing bowl, mix together the sugar, margarine, egg substitute, molasses, and warm water. Blend in the remaining cookie ingredients (the dough will be fairly thin). Cover the bowl and refrigerate the dough for at least 1 hour.

Drop by the rounded teaspoonful onto ungreased cookie sheets. Bake for about 8 minutes. Immediately remove the cookies from the baking sheets to cool on wire racks.

Frost the cookies after they've cooled.

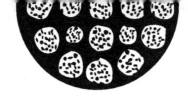

Monogrammed Cookies

Yield: 72 cookies, each with: Calories: 63 • Saturated Fat: 0.54 g • Total Fat: 3.21 g • Cholesterol: 0.02 mg

Now you can personalize your cookies! These are a light roll-and-cut sugar cookie, with a hint of almond flavor.

1 cup sugar
1 cup tub-style margarine, at room temperature
3 tablespoons skim milk
¼ cup egg substitute (see page 6)
1 teaspoon almond extract
3 cups all-purpose flour
1½ teaspoons baking powder
¼ teaspoon salt
1 teaspoon water
¼ cup egg substitute (see page 6)
Food coloring

Preheat the oven to 400° F.

In a large mixing bowl, cream together the sugar, margarine, and milk; add the ¼ cup egg substitute and the almond extract; mix well. Stir in the flour, baking powder, and salt; blend thoroughly. Divide the dough in half, form each half into a ball, and chill for at least 30 minutes.

On a lightly floured surface, roll out the dough, half of it at a time, to a ¼-inch thickness. Cut out shapes with floured cookie cutters, and place the cookies 1 inch apart on an ungreased cookie sheet.

To personalize your cookies, mix the water with the remaining ¼ cup egg substitute; stir well. Separate the egg mixture into 4 custard cups, and to each cup add 1 to 2 drops of a different color food coloring. With a clean, small artist brush, paint each cookie with the design or name of your choice. (Use a brush with synthetic bristles, as natural bristles may contain dormant bacteria.) Place the cookie sheet in the preheated oven and bake for 5 to 8 minutes. Immediately remove the cookies from the baking sheets to cool on wire racks.

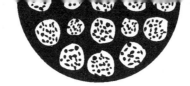

Rolled Oat Cookies

◆◆

Yield: 24 cookies, each with: Calories: 67 • Saturated Fat: 0.5 g • Total Fat: 2.97 g • Cholesterol: 0.01 mg

This thin, crisp cookie is a delightful variation on the traditional oatmeal raisin cookie. They are delicious plain or frosted with Buttercream Icing (page 170).

1 cup whole wheat pastry flour
¼ teaspoon salt
1 teaspoon baking powder
⅓ cup tub-style margarine
1 cup rolled oats
3 tablespoons light brown sugar
3 tablespoons white sugar
¼ cup egg substitute (see page 6)
2 teaspoons water

Preheat the oven to 350° F.

In a large bowl, sift together the flour, salt, and baking powder. Cut in the margarine with a fork or pastry blender. Add the oats and sugars, and mix well. Add the egg substitute and water; blend well.

Knead the dough into a smooth ball and place on a well-floured pastry cloth. Roll to a ¼-inch thickness and cut into your favorite shapes with a cookie cutter. Bake on ungreased cookie sheets for 20 minutes, or until very lightly browned. Immediately remove from the baking sheets to cool completely on wire racks.

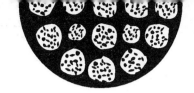

Honey Cookies

◆◆

Yield: 48 cookies, each with: Calories: 64 • Saturated Fat: 0.23 g • Total Fat: 1.4 g • Cholesterol: 0.01 mg

Christmas baking would not be complete at our house without these unique Honey Cookies, which are always a favorite for decorating.

⅓ cup tub-style margarine, at room
    temperature
⅓ cup packed light brown sugar
¼ cup egg substitute (see page 6)
⅔ cup honey
2⅔ cups all-purpose flour
1 teaspoon baking soda
½ teaspoon salt
1 teaspoon vanilla extract
1 cup powdered sugar
Small amount of milk

Preheat the oven to 350° F. Grease 2 baking sheets with tub-style margarine or spray with vegetable oil.

In a large mixing bowl, blend together the margarine, brown sugar, egg substitute, and honey. (If you rinse the liquid measuring cup with hot tap water before measuring the honey, the honey will slip right out.) Mix the honey mixture well. Stir in the flour, baking soda, and salt. Add the vanilla and blend thoroughly. Gather the dough into a ball and chill for 1 hour.

On a floured surface, roll the dough to a ¼-inch thickness. Cut it into shapes with a cookie cutter. Place cookies on the baking sheets, and bake for 8 to 10 minutes. Immediately remove the cookies from the baking sheets to cool completely on wire racks.

147

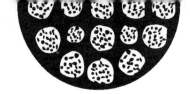

Fig Cookies

◆◆

Yield: 36 cookies, each with: Calories: 80 • Saturated Fat: 0.47 g • Total Fat: 2.84 g • Cholesterol: 0.02 mg

These are favorites of my father, who has always appreciated many of the finer things in life—his family, the perfect putting green, and freshly picked figs!

½ cup tub-style margarine, at room
    temperature
1 cup packed light brown sugar
½ cup egg substitute (see page 6)
2 tablespoons non-fat plain yogurt
1 cup chopped fresh figs
1 cup whole wheat flour
1¼ cups all-purpose flour
½ teaspoon cinnamon
1 teaspoon baking soda

Preheat the oven to 350° F. Grease 2 baking sheets with tub-style margarine or spray with vegetable oil.

In a large mixing bowl, blend together the margarine, brown sugar, and egg substitute; beat for 2 minutes at medium speed. Add the yogurt and the figs, and beat for another minute. Add the flours, cinnamon, and baking soda; mix well. Gather the dough into a ball and chill for 1 hour.

On a lightly floured surface, roll out the dough to a ⅛-inch thickness. Cut the dough with a cookie cutter. Bake the cookies on the baking sheets for 10 to 12 minutes. Immediately remove the cookies from the baking sheets to cool completely on wire racks.

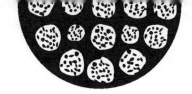

Poppy Seed Spice Cookies

Yield: 36 cookies, each with: Calories: 102 • Saturated Fat: 0.73 g • Total Fat: 4.32 g • Cholesterol: 0.03 mg

Keeping our cookie jar full is a never-ending joy to me. I try to keep a supply of favorites in the jar, ones like these rolled cookies that are so full of flavor.

¾ **cup tub-style margarine, at room temperature**
¾ **cup packed light brown sugar**
½ **cup white sugar**
1 **tablespoon vanilla extract**
½ **cup egg substitute (see page 6)**
3 **tablespoons skim milk**
3 **cups all-purpose flour**
1½ **teaspoons baking powder**
½ **teaspoon salt**
1 **teaspoon nutmeg**
1 **teaspoon cinnamon**
2 **tablespoons poppy seeds**

Preheat the oven to 350° F.

In a large mixing bowl, combine the margarine, sugars, and vanilla. Beat for 2 minutes at medium speed. Add the egg substitute and milk; blend well. Add the flour, baking powder, salt, spices, and poppy seeds. Blend thoroughly. Gather the dough into a ball, cover, and refrigerate for 1 hour.

On a floured surface, roll out the dough to a ¼-inch thickness and cut with a cookie cutter. Bake on ungreased baking sheets for 10 to 12 minutes. Cool the cookies on the pan for 1 minute before removing from the baking sheets to finish cooling on wire racks.

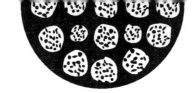

Anise Biscotti

Yield: 28 cookies, each with: Calories: 93 • Saturated Fat: 0.41 g • Total Fat: 2.92 g • Cholesterol: 0.02 mg

Biscotti—twice-baked cookies—are great with after-dinner coffee or tea. They'll keep for up to 2 weeks in an airtight container.

³⁄₄ **cup egg substitute (see page 6)**
³⁄₄ **cup granulated sugar**
¼ **cup tub-style margarine, melted**
2 **cups all-purpose flour**
2 **teaspoons baking powder**
2 **teaspoons anise extract**
1 **cup powdered sugar**
2 **to 3 teaspoons water**
½ **cup sliced almonds, toasted**

Preheat the oven to 350° F. Grease 2 baking sheets.

Beat together the egg substitute and sugar. Add the margarine, flour, baking powder, and anise extract; mix thoroughly.

Divide the dough in half. Spread each half into a 14-inch by 4-inch by 1-inch rectangle on a baking sheet. Bake for 20 minutes, or until golden brown. Quickly cut on the diagonal into 1-inch-thick biscuits. Lay the biscuits down on the same baking sheet and broil for 2 to 3 minutes, or until browned on the edges. Remove from the oven and cool on wire racks.

Mix the powdered sugar with the water until it's the consistency of frosting. Frost each biscuit and sprinkle with almonds.

150

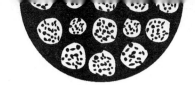

Cocoa Fudge Brownies

Yield: 12 brownies, each with: Calories: 200 • Saturated Fat: 1.27 g • Total Fat: 11.3 g • Cholesterol: 0.02 mg

These are very fudgy and chewy, delicious with an ice-cold glass of milk.

⅔ cup all-purpose flour
½ teaspoon baking powder
¼ teaspoon salt
1 tablespoon instant non-fat dry milk
6 tablespoons unsweetened cocoa
   powder
1 cup sugar
⅓ cup safflower oil
½ cup water
2 egg whites, beaten until frothy
¾ cup chopped nuts

Preheat the oven to 325° F. Grease and lightly flour a 9-inch square baking dish.

In a large mixing bowl, combine the flour, baking powder, salt, instant milk, cocoa, and sugar. Add the safflower oil and water, and beat at medium speed until smooth. Fold in the beaten egg whites and nuts. Pour the batter into the baking dish. Bake for 35 to 40 minutes, or until the brownies feel firm to the touch. Cut into squares while still slightly warm.

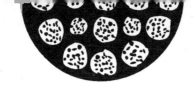

Butterscotch Treats

Yield: 9 bar cookies, each with: Calories: 218 • Saturated Fat: 0.96 g • Total Fat: 10.6 g • Cholesterol: 0.21 mg

Similar in texture to brownies, this toffee bar cookie is a great traveler.

⅔ cup sifted cake flour
¼ teaspoon salt
1 teaspoon baking powder
1 cup packed dark brown sugar
¼ cup safflower oil
¼ cup egg substitute (see page 6)
1 teaspoon vanilla extract
½ cup chopped walnuts

Preheat the oven to 350° F. Grease an 8-inch square baking pan with tub-style margarine.

Sift together the cake flour, salt, and baking powder. Set aside.

In a large mixing bowl, mix the brown sugar and safflower oil; blend until smooth. Add the egg substitute and vanilla to the sugar and oil mixture, and beat until light and fluffy. Stir in the nuts, then fold in the flour mixture.

Spread the batter in the prepared baking pan and bake for 35 minutes. Cool the brownies in the pan on a wire rack before cutting into bars.

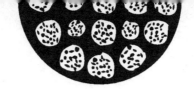

Apple Blondies

❖❖

Yield: 9 bar cookies, each with: Calories: 276 • Saturated Fat: 2.18 g • Total Fat: 14.9 g • Cholesterol: 0.02 g

This old-fashioned bar cookie, thick with fresh fruit and nuts, is always a favorite.

½ **cup tub-style margarine, at room temperature**
2 egg whites
¼ **cup egg substitute (see page 6)**
¾ **cup sugar**
3 apples, pared and diced
½ **cup chopped walnuts**
1 cup all-purpose flour
½ **teaspoon baking powder**
½ **teaspoon baking soda**
½ **teaspoon cinnamon**

Preheat the oven to 350° F. Grease an 8-inch square baking pan with tub-style margarine and dust lightly with flour.

In a large mixing bowl, cream together the margarine, egg whites, egg substitute, and sugar. Stir in the apples. Mix together the walnuts, flour, baking powder, baking soda, and cinnamon. Add to the creamed mixture, and blend well. Pour into the prepared baking pan. Bake for 40 minutes, or until a wooden pick inserted in the center comes out clean. Cool before cutting into squares.

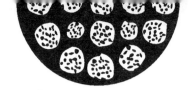

Applesauce Cake Bars

Yield: 18 squares, each with: Calories: 208 • Saturated Fat: 1.30 mg • Total Fat: 9.56 g • Cholesterol: 0.01 mg

These cookies travel well.

½ cup tub-style margarine, at room
    temperature
¾ cup granulated sugar
¼ cup egg substitute (see page 6)
1 teaspoon vanilla extract
1 cup sliced dates
1 cup coarsely chopped walnuts
1½ cups unsweetened applesauce
½ teaspoon cinnamon
¼ teaspoon cloves
2 cups all-purpose flour, sifted
2 teaspoons baking soda
2 tablespoons powdered sugar

Preheat the oven to 350° F. Grease a 9-inch by 13-inch baking pan with tub-style margarine and lightly dust with flour.

In a large mixing bowl, cream together the margarine and granulated sugar. Add the egg substitute and vanilla, and mix well. Blend in the dates, walnuts, and applesauce. Add the spices, flour, and baking soda; mix thoroughly.

Spread the batter in the prepared baking pan and bake for 20 minutes. Remove from the oven and cool on a wire rack before cutting into squares. Dust with powdered sugar.

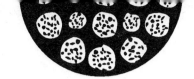

Almond Bar Cookies

❖❖

Yield: 20 squares, each with: Calories: 138 • Saturated Fat: 1.33 g • Total Fat: 3.36 g • Cholesterol: 0 mg

My six-year-old loves to help make these buttery, shortbread cookies; he has a flair for arranging the almonds over the top.

³/₄ cup tub-style margarine, at room
    temperature
½ cup sugar
2 cups all-purpose flour
1 tablespoon grated blanched almonds
¼ teaspoon salt
¼ cup blanched whole almonds

Preheat the oven to 325° F.

In a large mixing bowl, beat together the margarine and sugar. Add the flour, grated almonds, and salt. Mix until the dough is smooth. Press the dough into a rectangle shape (about 14 inches by 6 inches by ¼ inch) on an ungreased baking sheet. Arrange the whole almonds in rows over the top. Bake for 30 minutes. Remove from the oven and cut into 2-inch squares while still hot. Cool the bars completely on the baking sheet before removing.

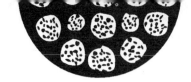

Date Squares

❖❖❖

Yield: 16 squares, each with: Calories: 238 • Saturated Fat: 1.62 g • Total Fat: 9.38 g • Cholesterol: 0 mg

This rich but not oversweet bar cookie resembles a crisp with its crumbly baked topping.

8 ounces pitted dates, coarsely chopped
1 cup orange juice
2 cups rolled oats
1 cup all-purpose flour
¾ cup packed light brown sugar
¼ cup white sugar
¼ teaspoon cinnamon
1 teaspoon baking soda
¾ cup tub-style margarine, melted

Preheat the oven to 350° F. Grease a 9-inch square baking pan with tub-style margarine or spray with vegetable oil.

In a small saucepan, simmer the dates and orange juice for 25 minutes, or until thick.

Stir together the oats, flour, sugars, cinnamon, and baking soda in a medium-size mixing bowl. Add the melted margarine, and stir until the mixture is crumbly.

Press half of the oat mixture in the bottom of the prepared baking pan. Spread the date mixture evenly over this, and sprinkle the remaining oat mixture on top. Bake for 45 minutes. Cool completely on a wire rack before cutting into squares.

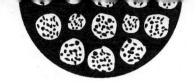

Cranberry Date Bars

Yield: 24 bars, each with: Calories: 237 • Saturated Fat: 1.42 g • Total Fat: 8.22 g • Cholesterol: 0 mg

This three-layer bar cookie is filled with the sweet and tart combination of dates and fresh cranberries.

1 (12-ounce) package cranberries
1 (8-ounce) package chopped, pitted dates
½ cup water
1 teaspoon vanilla extract
2 cups all-purpose flour
2 cups rolled oats
1¼ cups packed light brown sugar
½ teaspoon baking soda
¼ teaspoon salt
1 cup tub-style margarine, melted
Orange Glaze (page 172)

Preheat the oven to 350° F.

Combine the cranberries, dates, and water in a medium-size saucepan. Cook, covered, over low heat for 10 to 15 minutes, or until the cranberries pop, stirring frequently. Stir in the vanilla; set aside.

In a bowl, combine the flour, rolled oats, brown sugar, baking soda, and salt. Stir in the margarine until well blended.

Pat half of the oat mixture into an ungreased 9-inch by 13-inch baking pan. Bake for 8 minutes. Remove from the oven, and carefully spread the filling over the top. Sprinkle the remaining oat mixture on top, patting carefully. Bake for 20 minutes, or until golden brown. Cool on a wire rack. Drizzle the glaze over the cookies before cutting into bars.

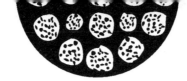

Frosted Banana Yogurt Bars

◆◆◆

Yield: 24 bars, each with: Calories: 210 • Saturated Fat: 1.2 g • Total Fat: 7.7 g • Cholesterol: 0.11 mg

Topped with Browned Butter Frosting, this single-layer bar cookie tastes like banana cake.

1½ cups sugar
1 (8-ounce) carton non-fat plain yogurt
½ cup tub-style margarine, at room
　temperature
½ cup egg substitute (see page 6)
1½ cups mashed bananas (about 3 large
　bananas)
2 teaspoons vanilla extract
2 cups all-purpose flour
1 teaspoon salt
1 teaspoon baking soda
½ cup chopped walnuts
Browned Butter Frosting (page 173)

Preheat the oven to 375° F. Grease a 10-inch by 15½-inch jelly roll pan with tub-style margarine and lightly dust with flour.

In a large mixing bowl, combine the sugar, yogurt, margarine, and egg substitute and beat on low speed for 1 minute. Add the bananas and vanilla and beat for another 30 seconds. Beat in the flour, salt, and baking soda on medium speed for another minute, scraping the bowl occasionally. Stir in the nuts. Spread the dough in the jelly roll pan and bake for 20 to 25 minutes, or until lightly browned. Cool completely on a wire rack.

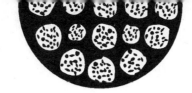

Frosted Zucchini Bars

Yield: 36 bars, each with: Calories: 123 • Saturated Fat: 0.93 g • Total Fat: 6.23 g • Cholesterol: 0.02 mg

I cut these tender and cake-like bar cookies into diamond shapes. To do this, first make straight parallel cuts 1 to 1½ inches apart down the length of the pan. Then make diagonal cuts in the opposite direction.

1¾ cups all-purpose flour
1½ teaspoons baking powder
¾ cup tub-style margarine, at room temperature
½ cup white sugar
½ cup packed light brown sugar
½ cup egg substitute (see page 6)
1 teaspoon vanilla extract
2 cups grated zucchini
¾ cup chopped walnuts
Cinnamon Frosting (page 173)

Preheat the oven to 350° F. Grease a 10-inch by 15½-inch jelly roll pan with tub-style margarine.

In a small mixing bowl, stir together the flour and baking powder; set aside.

In a large mixing bowl, beat the margarine and sugars for 1 minute on medium speed. Add the egg substitute and vanilla, and blend well. Stir in the flour mixture, zucchini, and walnuts. Spread evenly in the prepared baking pan and bake for 30 minutes, or until a wooden pick inserted in the center comes out clean. Cool completely in the pan on a wire rack. Drizzle the frosting on top before cutting into bars.

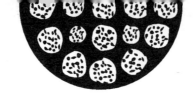

Black Forest Bars

❖❖

Yield: 16 servings, each with: Calories: 136 • Saturated Fat: 0.9 g • Total Fat: 4.71 g • Cholesterol: 0.03 mg

These have a chocolate base and a topping that is rich and gooey.

⅓ cup tub-style margarine, at room temperature
⅔ cup sugar
⅔ cup egg substitute (see page 6)
1 teaspoon vanilla extract
⅔ cup all-purpose flour
⅓ cup unsweetened cocoa powder
½ teaspoon baking powder
¼ teaspoon salt
1 (20-ounce) can cherry pie filling
2 egg whites
⅛ teaspoon cream of tartar
2 tablespoons sugar
¼ teaspoon vanilla extract

Preheat the oven to 325° F. Grease a 9-inch by 13-inch baking pan with tub-style margarine.

Cream the margarine; add the sugar, beating well at medium speed. Add the egg substitute and 1 teaspoon of the vanilla; beat well. Add the flour, cocoa, baking powder, and salt; stir well.

Spread the batter in the prepared baking dish and bake for 18 minutes. Cool completely in the pan.

Preheat the oven to 450° F.

Spread the pie filling evenly over the cake.

Beat the egg whites and the cream of tartar at high speed until soft peaks form. Gradually add the 2 tablespoons of sugar,

160

beating until stiff peaks form. Fold in the remaining ¼ teaspoon vanilla. Spoon the mixture into a decorating bag fitted with a large star tip, and pipe 16 meringue dollops onto the pie filling. Bake for 8 minutes, or until the meringue is lightly browned. Cut into 16 squares after the bars have cooled.

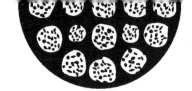

Apple Butter Oatmeal Bars

Yield: 24 bars, each with: Calories: 106 • Saturated Fat: 0.86 g • Total Fat: 5.78 g • Cholesterol: 0.01 mg

½ cup tub-style margarine, at room temperature
½ cup packed light brown sugar
¼ cup egg substitute (see page 6)
½ cup sweetened apple butter
⅔ cup all-purpose flour
½ teaspoon baking powder
½ teaspoon baking soda
¼ teaspoon salt
1 cup rolled oats
½ cup chopped walnuts
2 tablespoons powdered sugar

Preheat the oven to 350° F. Grease a 9-inch by 13-inch baking pan with tub-style margarine.

In a large mixing bowl, beat the margarine and brown sugar until light and fluffy. Add the egg substitute and apple butter; blend well. Add the flour, baking powder, baking soda, and salt. Beat until well blended. Stir in the oats and chopped nuts. Spread the batter in the prepared pan, and bake for 15 to 20 minutes. Sift powdered sugar over the top while still warm. Cool on a wire rack before cutting into bars.

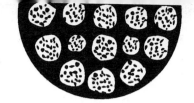

Butterscotch-Meringue Bar

Yield: 16 bars, each with: Calories: 251 • Saturated Fat: 1.42 g • Total Fat: 9.74 g • Cholesterol: 0.03 mg

Pastry

½ cup tub-style margarine, at room
    temperature
1 cup white sugar
½ cup egg substitute (see page 6)
1 teaspoon vanilla extract
1½ cups all-purpose flour
½ teaspoon salt
1 teaspoon baking powder

Meringue

1 egg white
1 cup packed light brown sugar
½ cup chopped walnuts

Preheat the oven to 375° F. Grease a 9-inch by 13-inch baking pan with tub-style margarine.

In a medium-size mixing bowl, cream the margarine; add the white sugar and mix well. Add the egg substitute and vanilla; blend together. Add the flour, salt, and baking powder; continue beating for 2 minutes. Spread the batter in the prepared baking pan.

To prepare the meringue layer, beat the egg white at high speed until stiff in a small mixing bowl. Add the brown sugar and continue to beat until stiff. Fold in the chopped nuts. Spread the meringue evenly over the pastry layer. Bake for 25 minutes. Cool the cookies in the pan before cutting into bars.

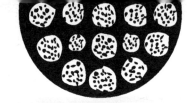

Meringues

❖❖

Yield: 36 meringues, each with: Calories: 23 • Saturated Fat: 0 g • Total Fat: 0 g • Cholesterol: 0 mg

Meringues are always a favorite with children, as they melt like magic in their mouths. The secret to making meringues is the timing—work quickly so the meringue doesn't wilt.

4 egg whites
1 cup sugar
1 teaspoon vanilla extract
Dash salt

Preheat the oven to 250° F. Line 2 baking sheets with parchment or waxed paper.

In a small mixing bowl, beat the egg whites until stiff but not dry. Add the sugar, vanilla, and salt; mix well. Drop by the teaspoonful, about 1 inch apart, onto the baking sheets. Bake for 1½ hours. The meringues should be quite dry but still slightly chewy inside. Cool on wire racks.

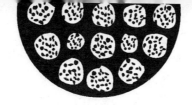

Pecan Kisses

◆◆

Yield: 54 meringues, each with: Calories: 46 • Saturated Fat: 0.24 • Total Fat: 2.98 g • Cholesterol: 0 mg

Experiment with different extracts for this meringue cookie. Equal parts of vanilla and orange extracts also produce a delightful flavor.

6 egg whites
1 cup sugar
½ teaspoon cream of tartar
1 teaspoon vanilla extract
2 cups coarsely chopped pecans

Preheat the oven to 300° F. Line 2 baking sheets with parchment or waxed paper.

In a large mixing bowl, beat 1 egg white until stiff. Gradually add 2 tablespoons of sugar. Add another egg white, continuing to beat constantly, then add another 2 tablespoons sugar. Continue this until all the egg whites and 12 tablespoons of sugar are added. Mix the remaining 4 tablespoons sugar with the cream of tartar, and gradually add this to the egg whites, beating until very stiff. Fold in the vanilla and nuts.

Drop by the teaspoonful 1 inch apart onto the baking sheets. Bake for 25 minutes. The cookies should be cracked on top, but not browned. Cool on wire racks.

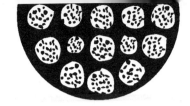

Cocoa Meringues

❖❖❖

Yield: 15 large meringues, each with: Calories: 58 • Saturated Fat: 0.23 g • Total Fat: 1.38 g • Cholesterol: 0 mg

The inside of this meringue tastes like a fudge brownie. These are also delicious if you omit the slivered almonds and instead top each with a pecan half.

3 egg whites
⅛ teaspoon cream of tartar
¾ cup sugar
3 tablespoons unsweetened cocoa powder
½ teaspoon vanilla extract
¼ cup slivered almonds

Preheat the oven to 325° F. Line 2 baking sheets with parchment or waxed paper.

In a small mixing bowl, beat the egg whites and cream of tartar at high speed until stiff peaks form. Gradually add the sugar, beating well until shiny. Add the cocoa and vanilla; blend well. Fold in the almonds.

Drop by the tablespoonful 3 inches apart onto the baking sheets. Bake for 25 minutes. The meringues should be crisp on the outside. Remove and cool on wire racks.

7
Sauces, Frostings, and Icings

In this chapter, you will find recipes for toppings and frostings for cakes and cookies. The nutritional analyses for the fruit sauces are given per serving, but the analyses for the frostings, icings, and glazes are given for the entire recipe.

Sweet Cherry Sauce

This makes a perfect topping for angel food cake. In a medium-size saucepan, combine 1½ pounds fresh or canned pitted sweet cherries, ½ cup white grape juice, 2½ teaspoons lemon juice, ½ teaspoon almond extract, and 1 teaspoon lemon zest. Cook over medium low heat for 35 to 40 minutes, stirring frequently, until slightly thickened. Remove from the heat and stir in 2 teaspoons sugar and ½ cup toasted chopped almonds. Yield: 10 servings (2½ cups) • Calories: 101 • Saturated Fat: 0.44 g • Total Fat: 4.23 g • Cholesterol: 0 mg.

Strawberry Sauce

Great to top pound cake and angel food cake. In a small saucepan, combine a 12-ounce jar of low-sugar strawberry preserves with ½ cup orange juice and 1 tablespoon orange rind strips. Heat over low heat just until the preserves melt. Remove from the heat and stir in 1 pint fresh or frozen strawberries, hulled and sliced. The sauce can be stored in the refrigerator for up to a week. Yield: 12 servings • Calories: 87 • Saturated Fat: 0.006 g • Total Fat: 0.13 g • Cholesterol: 0 mg.

Blueberry Sauce

Excellent on top of pound cake and angel food cake. In a medium-size saucepan, mix together 2 cups fresh or frozen blueberries, ⅓ cup sugar, and 1 tablespoon lemon juice. Cook over medium heat, stirring and crushing the blueberries a little. Bring the mixture to a boil; boil for 1 minute. Remove from the heat and stir in ½ teaspoon vanilla extract. Cool. Store leftover sauce in the refrigerator. Yield: 8 servings (2 cups) • Calories: 53 • Saturated Fat: 0.01 g • Total Fat: 0.14 g • Cholesterol: 0 mg.

Fudge Frosting

In a medium-size saucepan, stir together 3 tablespoons unsweetened cocoa powder, 1 cup sugar, and ¼ teaspoon salt. Stir in ⅓ cup evaporated skim milk and 3 tablespoons safflower oil. Bring to a boil over medium heat, stirring occasionally. Reduce the heat to simmer and cook for another 1 to 2 minutes. Remove from the heat; add 1 teaspoon vanilla. Beat by hand for 5 minutes, or until smooth and of spreading consistency. Yield: Frosting for a 2-layer cake or a 9-inch by 13-inch sheet cake • Calories: 1240 • Saturated Fat: 5.58 g • Total Fat: 44.1 g • Cholesterol: 3.33 mg.

Brown Sugar Frosting

Combine ¼ cup water and 1 cup packed dark brown sugar in a medium-size saucepan and cook until the soft ball stage (234° F. on a candy thermometer) stage is reached. Remove from the heat. In a small mixing bowl, beat 2 egg whites and ¼ teaspoon cream of tartar until foamy, then gradually add the sugar syrup. Continue beating at high speed until the frosting is cool and stiff.

Yield: Frosting for a 2-layer cake or a 9-inch by 13-inch sheet cake • Calories: 855 • Saturated Fat: 0 g • Total Fat: 0 g • Cholesterol: 0 mg

Fluffy White Frosting

In a small mixing bowl, beat 3 egg whites, a dash of salt, a dash of cream of tartar, and $\frac{1}{4}$ cup sugar until glossy. Beat in $\frac{3}{4}$ cup light corn syrup very slowly, until the mixture is very fluffy. Add 1 teaspoon vanilla and blend well. Yield: Frosting for a 2-layer cake or a 9-inch by 13-inch sheet cake • Calories: 928 • Saturated Fat: 0 g • Total Fat: 0 g • Cholesterol: 0 mg.

Buttercream Icing

Blend $\frac{1}{4}$ cup tub-style margarine with 2 cups powdered sugar. Beat in 1 tablespoon skim milk and 1 teaspoon vanilla extract until the frosting is of spreading consistency. Yield: Frosting for 48 cookies or 1 angel food cake • Calories: 1200 • Saturated Fat: 7.66 g • Total Fat: 45.6 g • Cholesterol: 0.48 mg.

Chocolate Buttercream Icing

Blend together $\frac{1}{4}$ cup tub-style margarine, $1\frac{3}{4}$ cups powdered sugar, dash salt, $\frac{1}{4}$ cup unsweetened cocoa powder, and 2 tablespoons skim milk. Beat until smooth. Stir in $\frac{1}{2}$ teaspoon vanilla extract. Yield: Frosting for 48 cookies • Calories: 1152 • Saturated Fat: 10.08 g • Total Fat: 49.9 g • Cholesterol: 0.48 mg.

170

Vanilla Glaze

Excellent on angel food cake and spice cupcakes. In a small mixing bowl, beat 2 egg whites at medium speed until foamy. Gradually add ¾ cup powdered sugar, beating until well blended. Mix in 1 teaspoon lemon juice, ¼ teaspoon cream of tartar, and another ¾ cup powdered sugar. Continue beating until the glaze is thick. Yield: Frosting for a 2-layer cake or a 9-inch by 13-inch sheet cake • Calories: 613 • Saturated Fat: 0.002 g • Total Fat: 0.02 g • Cholesterol: 0 mg.

Chocolate Meringue Frosting

In a medium-size saucepan over low heat, stir together 1 cup packed light brown sugar and ½ cup water. Bring to a boil and continue cooking until the syrup spins a thread (230° F.). In a small mixing bowl, beat 2 egg whites until stiff. Pour the syrup mixture over the egg whites and mix until smooth and stiff enough to spread. Stir in ¼ cup unsweetened cocoa powder and ½ teaspoon vanilla extract. Yield: Frosting for a 2-layer cake or a 9-inch by 13-inch sheet cake • Calories: 910 • Saturated Fat: 2.35 g • Total Fat: 4.07 g • Cholesterol: 0 mg.

Mocha Icing

Stir together 3 tablespoons unsweetened cocoa powder and 3 tablespoons strong, hot decaffeinated coffee. Add ½ teaspoon vanilla extract and 1½ cups powdered sugar and beat by hand until the icing is smooth and easy to spread. Yield: Frosting for a 2-layer cake or a 9-inch by 13-inch sheet cake • Calories: 620 • Saturated Fat: 1.76 g • Total Fat: 3.06 g • Cholesterol: 0 mg.

Creamy Pineapple Frosting

In a small mixing bowl, combine 4 cups powdered sugar with 6 tablespoons softened tub-style margarine on low speed until well mixed. Add ½ cup well-drained crushed pineapple and beat until fluffy. If needed, add additional powdered sugar to make the frosting a good spreading consistency. Yield: Frosting for a 2-layer cake or a 9-inch by 13-inch sheet cake • Calories: 2188 • Saturated Fat: 111.8 g • Total Fat: 69 g • Cholesterol: 0 mg.

Orange Glaze Icing

Blend together 1½ tablespoons tub-style margarine and ¾ cup powdered sugar. Stir in 1 teaspoon grated orange rind, 1½ teaspoons orange juice, and ⅛ teaspoon vanilla. Beat until smooth and of spreading consistency. Yield: Frosting for 24 cookies • Calories: 446 • Saturated Fat: 2.94 g • Total Fat: 17.2 g • Cholesterol: 0 mg.

Orange Glaze

Stir together 2 cups sifted powdered sugar, 3 tablespoons orange juice, and ½ teaspoon vanilla extract until smooth. Yield: Frosting for 9-inch by 13-inch sheet cake or cookie bar • Calories: 791 • Saturated Fat: 0.01 g • Total Fat: 0.09 g • Cholesterol: 0 mg.

Browned Butter Frosting

Heat ¼ cup tub-style margarine over medium heat until a delicate brown; remove from the heat. Mix in 2 cups powdered sugar. Beat in 3 tablespoons skim milk and 1 teaspoon vanilla extract until smooth and of spreading consistency. Yield: Frosting for 9-inch by 13-inch sheet cake or cookie bar • Calories: 1193 • Saturated Fat: 7.88 g • Total Fat: 45.8 g • Cholesterol: 0.75 mg.

Cinnamon Frosting

Melt 2 tablespoons tub-style margarine. Beat together the margarine, 2 cups powdered sugar, 2 tablespoons skim milk, 1 teaspoon cinnamon, ⅛ teaspoon nutmeg, and 1 teaspoon vanilla extract until smooth and of spreading consistency. Yield: Frosting for 9-inch by 13-inch sheet cake or 10-inch by 15½-inch cookie bar • Calories: 991 • Saturated Fat: 4.04 g • Total Fat: 23.1 g • Cholesterol: 0.5 mg.

Index

OTHER SPECIALTY COOKBOOKS FROM THE CROSSING PRESS

SAUCES FOR PASTA! By Kristie Trabant	$8.95	**SUN-DRIED TOMATOES!** By Andrea Chesman	$8.95
PESTOS! By Dorothy Rankin	$8.95	**SALSAS!** By Andrea Chesman	$8.95
PASTA SALADS! By Susan Janine Meyer	$8.95	**GOOD FOR YOU COOKIES!** By Jane Marsh Dieckmann	$8.95
SALAD DRESSINGS! By Jane Marsh Dieckmann	$8.95	**OLD WORLD BREADS!** By Charel Steele	$8.95
FRUIT DESSERTS! By Dorothy Parker	$8.95	**SORBETS!** By Jim Tarantino	$8.95
FAST BREADS! By Howard Early and Glenda Morris	$8.95	**BROWNIES, BARS, AND BISCOTTI!** By Terri Henry	$8.95
CONDIMENTS! By Jay Solomon	$8.95	**SPOON DESSERTS!** By Lynn Nusom	$8.95

Available at your local bookstore, or write directly to The Crossing Press, P. O. Box 1048, Freedom, CA 95019. Please add $2.00 for postage on the first book, and $ .50 for each additional book. If you wish, you may use VISA or MASTERCARD. Please give your number and expiration date.

We publish many more cookbooks. Please write or call TOLL FREE 800/777-1048 for a free catalog.